THE ULTIMATE CHINESE MARTIAL ART

The Science of the Weaving Stance Bagua
64 Forms and its Wellness Applications

THE ULTIMATE CHINESE MARTIAL ART

The Science of the Weaving Stance Bagua 64 Forms and its Wellness Applications

Jun Feng Li
World Academic Society of Medical Qigong, China

Chun Yan Ge
Inner Martial Art Research Association of Singapore, Singapore

Tong Luo
Possehl Electronics, Vice President, Asia Sales

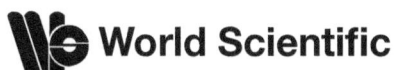

NEW JERSEY · LONDON · SINGAPORE · BEIJING · SHANGHAI · HONG KONG · TAIPEI · CHENNAI · TOKYO

Published by

World Scientific Publishing Co. Pte. Ltd.
5 Toh Tuck Link, Singapore 596224
USA office: 27 Warren Street, Suite 401-402, Hackensack, NJ 07601
UK office: 57 Shelton Street, Covent Garden, London WC2H 9HE

Library of Congress Cataloging-in-Publication Data
Names: Li, Jun Feng, author.
Title: The ultimate Chinese martial art : the science of the weaving stance bagua :
   64 forms and its wellness applications / Jun Feng Li, Chun Yan Ge, Tong Luo.
Description: Singapore : World Scientific, 2016.
Identifiers: LCCN 2016004863| ISBN 9789814749282 (hardcover : alk. paper) |
   ISBN 9814749281 (hardcover : alk. paper) | ISBN 9789814749299 (pbk. : alk. paper) |
   ISBN 981474929X (pbk. : alk. paper)
Subjects: LCSH: Martial arts--Health aspects. | Martial arts--Psychological aspects.
Classification: LCC GV1102.7.P75 L5 2016 | DDC 796.815/5--dc23
LC record available at https://lccn.loc.gov/2016004863

British Library Cataloguing-in-Publication Data
A catalogue record for this book is available from the British Library.

Copyright © 2017 by World Scientific Publishing Co. Pte. Ltd.

All rights reserved. This book, or parts thereof, may not be reproduced in any form or by any means, electronic or mechanical, including photocopying, recording or any information storage and retrieval system now known or to be invented, without written permission from the publisher.

For photocopying of material in this volume, please pay a copying fee through the Copyright Clearance Center, Inc., 222 Rosewood Drive, Danvers, MA 01923, USA. In this case permission to photocopy is not required from the publisher.

Contents

Prologue   vii

Part I   History and Philosophy of Chinese Martial Arts   1

Chapter 1   Taoism and Confucianism: Two Major Pillars of Chinese Rationalism   3
History of Taoism   4
A Few Key Things to Know and Remember About Taoism   6
Staying in the Middle of the Road: A Chinese Attitude of Facing the Unknown   16

Chapter 2   Further Development of Chinese Martial Arts   23
All Martial Arts Come from Shaolin-天下武功出少林   25
The Evolution from Outer School to Inner School   27
The Development of Bagua Palm As the Newest Traditional Chinese Martial Art   33

Chapter 3   How would Sir Isaac Newton Interpret Chinese Martial Arts: A New Scientific Approach to the Understanding of Chinese Martial Arts   39
Axiom 1: Force Is a Vector (The Σ: Direction Matters)   39
Axiom 2: $J = \Delta F/\Delta T$ (Jing is the Real Killer)   46
Axiom 3: The Δ and Σ Both Come from Your Liver   58

Part II Taoism in Action: The 64 Forms of Bagua Palm — 61

Chapter 4 Basic Principles for Practicing Bagua Palm — 65

Chapter 5 The Mud-Wading Steps — 79
Key Points for the Mud-Wading Steps — 81
A Detailed Illustration of Mud-Wading Steps — 83
First Step: Wading in a Straight Line Without Arm Movements — 84
Second Step: Circular Wading — 85
Third Step: Full Practice (Green Dragon Shows Claw) — 89
Appendix — 99

Chapter 6 The New 64 Forms of Weaving Stance Bagua Palm — 101
Brief Introduction — 101
List of the 64 Forms — 102
Starting Form — 104
Appendix I: Key Notes on Martial Art Training — 226

Part III The Applications of Bagua Palm — Physically and Mentally — 229

Chapter 7 A Basic Conflict in Our Life: How the Ultraslow Evolution of Our Body Cope with the Lightning-fast Changes of Our Environment — 231

Chapter 8 Anti-Fragile as a Concept and How Do We Understand "Strong"? — 241

Chapter 9 Outlive as a Target and the Martial Art Renaissance — 245

Epilogue — 251

Acknowledgments — 253

Prologue

From the Art of Killing to the Art of Outliving

Christians believe that we are all sinners. Biological evolution theory tells us that we are much worse: we are all killers.

Before agriculture was invented, there were no bankers, no lawyers, not even workers or farmers. All of us, like other creatures on this planet, survived as killers. We were either killing animals or killing each other. Except for plucking some low-hanging fruits occasionally, killing was the main way of getting food and thus one of mankind's major daily activities.

Killing is never about killing for its own sake, not even in ancient times. The reason man killed was mostly to survive. Man hunted and killed for food. Also, man killed in self-defense to eliminate a lethal threat, be it a tiger or another fighter from an enemy tribe.

As an art of killing, martial art was more than important. It was crucial. It was the key to food, sex, and security — the very basic human needs based on Maslow's hierarchy of needs. In more than 99% of human history, all men were fighters. That is the period when no actual history records existed.

During those millions of years when we were evolving, we were either fighting with animals or with other people when animals were hard to find. Those who did not fight well had little chance of having any descendants. Generation after generation, as the result of natural selection, men have been born great fighters. The human body has been physically designed and developed for fighting.

Even till very late in history before the appearance of guns, which was about 200 years ago, martial arts skill was crucial in the pursuit of power, which brings us to the next three elements in Maslow's hierarchy of needs — love/belonging, esteem, and self-actualization. That explains why knights occupied a higher social status in the western world and even in Japan, for a very long period of time in history.

The act of killing is always terrible. It is the worst but indispensable part of human history. However, according to Taoism, the best often comes from the worst. The martial arts are the ancient arts of killing, but people are starting to find the relevance of martial arts in modern life and are trying to apply what they learn from the martial arts to positive activities.

The next time you watch a wildlife documentary, observe the predators and their prey. Ninety-nine percent of the time, the predators are the calmer creatures. They lie idle on the ground and gaze around without much thinking. The prey are always nervous, easily spurred into a crazy run, sometimes even when there is no real threat.

On the other hand, even while not engaged in the killing process, the predators show more vitality than their prey. The same goes for martial artists. Martial artists usually look more calm and alive. This is a fresher angle to interpreting the art of outliving your peers — not just to live longer, but also to be more alive.

The martial arts, being such a crucial part of life, were bound to be studied diligently by many. The philosophy and methodology developed in the process of fine-tuning the art of killing have become an important part of a culture. Being very good in a martial art helps us to excel in other areas as well, because the basic philosophy behind the art is transferable. That is why a martial art is such a giant treasure trove where each of us can find something useful for our daily lives.

Now, let us start from the beginning.

Part I: History and Philosophy of Chinese Martial Arts

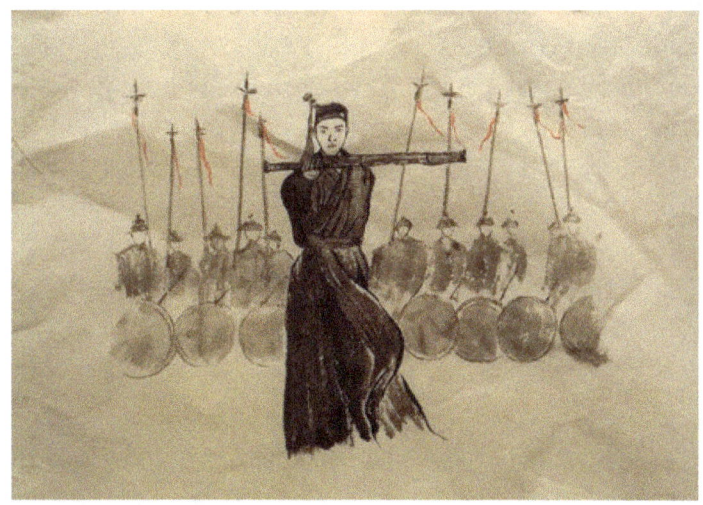

Nowadays, many people think of Chinese martial arts as being similar to dancing or gymnastics. If you watch many Chinese martial art competitions, it does appear to be so. However, the origins of Chinese martial art were more somber, being essentially for killing. It was no game. It was not even a sport.

Martial arts is not about jumping high or low, running fast or slow, being strong or weak, winning or losing, earning respect or contempt. Honor, pain, tears, and blood — all these are irrelevant to a Chinese *gongfu* master.

Chinese martial arts are arts of survival. They are only about life or death, nothing else.

In fact, if you really want to live, you cannot even afford to care too much about living or dying. Thinking too much about anything in a fight can only cost you your life.

Death can arrive at any point in time. Once it arrives, it cannot be undone, not like a computer game. That is why occasionally, a martial artist can look a bit too serious.

> I walk ahead and kill one enemy every 10 steps. After a thousand miles, still no one can stop me.
>
> Li Bai, *The Song for the Swordsmen*

This is the style of a real Chinese martial artist — ultimately unstoppable. In this sense, the Chinese martial art seems not much different from martial arts of other countries.

However, like all other martial arts from elsewhere in the world, Chinese martial arts have a unique approach influenced by local culture. The most important aspects of local culture for the Chinese are Taoism and Confucianism.

1
Taoism and Confucianism:
Two Major Pillars of Chinese Rationalism

It might seem strange to talk about an ancient Chinese religion at the very beginning of a martial arts book. The reason is both simple and complicated.

The simple part is the form we introduce in this book: Bagua, a Taoism-styled martial art. Actually, Bagua is the most thorough Taoism martial art that has ever appeared. From its name to its very core theory, it is all about Taoism.

The more complicated part is, Taoism is the root of all elements in typical Chinese culture, and that includes the Chinese martial arts as a whole, not just Bagua. Only with decent knowledge about Taoism can we understand the origin of Chinese martial arts.

At the same time, as a long-time "official" philosophy in China, Confucianism has such a vast influence on all aspects of Chinese culture and on many different trades, that we cannot talk about anything Chinese without a good understanding of Confucianism. In many cases, Confucianism and Taoism have mixed influences on trades such as calligraphy, painting, and even the Chinese medical system. Through Taoism and Confucianism, we also find connections of Chinese martial arts to all those trades.

Through studying the connections of Chinese martial arts to all the other seemingly irrelevant trades, we can gain a deeper understanding of the Chinese martial arts themselves. At the same time, such an understanding will enable us to find applications of what we learn from Chinese martial arts to all other aspects of our daily life.

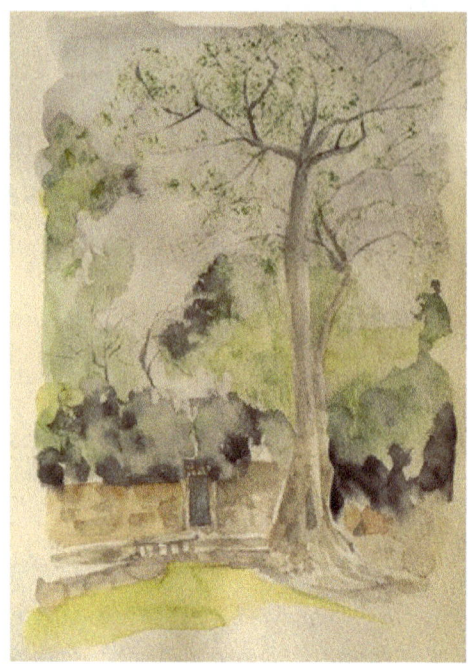

Fig. 1.1. Roots, trunk, and branches form the tree, and the different parts function as one.

The whole system is just like a tree. If the real martial art part is the trunk, Taoism and Confucianism are both its roots and branches. You do not want to paint a tree with only a trunk (Fig. 1.1).

This is also the learning style of a Chinese martial artist: to connect whatever you have learned from other subjects to martial arts and apply whatever you have learned in martial arts to all aspects of your daily life.

Simply put, if learning Chinese martial arts has not made you a better chef, driver, manager, banker, actor, singer, or calligrapher, you have not learned anything about Chinese martial arts.

Later we will explain further why this makes sense.

History of Taoism

In China, no religion has ever shown any dominance in normal people's daily lives. To be accurate, there has been actually no religion in China at all by western standards.

Very different from the situation in western society, people who devote themselves 100% to any religion are regarded by the Chinese as marginal people in society. People in China treat them as we treated gay people 20 years ago, largely because they have one thing in common: they do not reproduce.

This was also the case with the upper-class Chinese: Culturally, both Buddhism and Taoism have had an extensive influence on them, but more as a philosophical nutrition to their minds than as a placebo to their hearts.

The word *Tao* (道), which literally means *way*, came from the word *Dao* (蹈), which means *to step on*. In the early days of Chinese culture, all sorts of people called the methods of their trades *Tao*. The warriors called their methods *Wu Tao* (武道 the way of martial arts). The doctors called their trade *Yi Tao* (医道, the way of medical arts), etc.

Then why did only the Taoists in later years dominate the word Tao and call themselves Taoists? There is a reason for that. From the very beginning, Zhuang-zi (庄子) claimed that all the other trades are subjects with a different specific focus, while only Taoism covers the core wisdom of all those trades. It is like a wisdom about wisdom, which makes it a perfect match to philosophy rather than religion.

Buddhism was imported at a much later time, so Taoism as a home-grown "religion" had been virtually the only influential religion for a long time. As a home-grown religion, the Taoism approach represents the way Chinese interpret the world around them. Chinese martial arts are no exception. This is the major reason why we start from Taoism when we discuss Chinese martial arts.

At the same time, the Taoists, together with all other religious people in China, were regarded as 方外之士, which means people not involved in worldly affairs such as reproducing themselves. They had a much bigger degree of freedom to do whatever they wanted to. They also typically had more time to practice as they did not have social burdens, such as a family to support. So it is no surprise that many great fighters were Taoists or Buddhist monks, such as the legendary Wudang Clan and Shaolin monks.

Taoism was not a religion when Lao-zi and Zhuang-zi set the foundation of Taoism over 2000 years ago. Together with Confucianism, it is widely regarded as a school of philosophy that is essentially Chinese.

A Few Key Things to Know and Remember About Taoism

Few of us would plan to be scholars in Taoism. So we will only go through it briefly in this book. The good news is that, unlike a typical western philosophy, Taoism is not a complicated or complete system of interpreting everything around us. This makes it easier for us to present an "executive summary" of Taoism.

1. Taoism represents an inner-looking attitude toward everything.

First of all, Taoism does not believe in asking help from any form of supernatural external powers, be they gods or ghosts. Taoists do not encourage people to pray for their own benefit. They believe in *ji* (积 accumulate) *de* (德 good deeds). They believe they can make themselves gods if they do good deeds all the time and follow the right way to perfect themselves. It is almost a shame to ask help from God.

With that attitude, Taoists are more inner-looking than outer-looking in their focus. They tend to turn to themselves to find solutions to problems.

This attitude explains the important trait of the Taoism approach toward wellness: introspection. As Taoists do not believe in changing the nature of something with human efforts, they look more into themselves to find ways for wellness and many other things. It is very similar to Yoga, which focuses on awareness.

Small trick: Unlike a trained *gongfu* master, normal people do not feel the movement of blood or *Qi* (气, gas) inside their body. It is difficult then for them to actually be aware of their own body because they do not feel anything most of the time. That is why in the initial stage, lots of focus is on the breath. Anyone can feel the air going inside their body, and this feeling helps them to focus their mind in their own body, rather than focusing on, say, a bird flying over their head.

2. Taoism calls for respect toward nature and advocates being spontaneous rather than forceful.

The initial aim of Taoism looks simple: to live long with meaningful activeness.

However, despite all the attention on longevity, Lao-zi and Zhuang-zi did not believe in living as long as possible at all costs. (They were even at times critical of people devoting a lot of their time to doing exercises just for the sake of living longer.)

The main preaching of Taoism even as a religion is this: the Tao follows nature. What the Taoists or most Chinese are against is *ni* (逆 opposite) *tian* (天 heaven) which means to go against the laws of nature. You may call this a planter's philosophy, which typically handles things like a farmer dealing with the weather — making attempts to predict what is going on and acting accordingly to minimize damage and optimize gain.

The word *nature* in Chinese is a combination of two characters: *zi* (自 self) and *ran* (然: appearance, look like). So, for the Chinese, nature is just the way it is. It is not our business to change it. However, we can find whatever we need by watching the way nature runs itself. That is why we believe the Chinese are ardent students of nature. By observing all the different aspects of nature, we can know more about ourselves.

The most vivid explanation of this phrase comes from a famous article by Zhuang-zi.

In 《养生主》, an article about wellness, he told a story about a butcher who was frustrated by the fact that his knife became blunt easily after dismembering a bull.

He then spent three years to observe the structure of a bull until he was so familiar with it that he no longer saw a whole bull when he cut it — what he saw was only the joints of the animal. He could then place his knife to the soft joints and dismember the bull without much effort. As a result, his knife remained like new after 19 years dismembering thousands of bulls.

The moral of the story is: the best way toward wellness is to follow the way of nature. The essence is to respect the rules of nature, which is the ultimate pursuit of today's science.

In martial art terms, the Taoism approach is to be spontaneous and go with the flow rather than being forceful all the time. This results in quicker reactions with intuition in real fighting and less injuries in daily practice.

3. The core concept of Taoism is change.

The first sentence of the Taoism classic by Lao-zi says: "The way can be followed, but there is no such thing as a constant way." This can be interpreted as viewing the world we are in as an ever-changing object.

The world changes on its own and is not controlled by any external forces such as immortal creatures. The driver of change has to come from internal forces.

Change is a necessary element of life — a positive force to refresh our lives. This concept of change has deeply influenced the inner style of Chinese martial arts.

To illustrate the concept of ultimate change, many basic concepts were developed around it, such as *Yin* and *Yang*, Bagua, and the annoyingly omnipresent concept, *Qi*.

Yin and Yang: A Chinese Perspective of Change

Yin and *Yang* is a unique philosophical concept in Chinese culture. Initially, *Yin* was a simplified drawing of the moon and *Yang* of the sun, which were then used to represent night and day, and then further stretched to represent any pair of opposite characters or two contradictory status — dark and bright, cold and hot, etc.

In Chinese martial arts *Yin* and *Yang* can stand for soft and hard, hidden and obvious, or be as simple as two sides or your palm.

Yin and *Yang* have a separate status when used on their own. However, *Yin* and *Yang* combined is a concept or even a whole school of philosophy focused on the study of change.

The famous Chinese book <<易>> or *Book of Changes* is about change. The Chinese character *yi* (易) is formed by the sun and the moon (Fig. 1.2), both characterized by periodical change, a change that ancient Chinese somehow understood and were able to predict with great accuracy.

This scene is not difficult to imagine: if you were a hairy creature sitting in the woods 10,000 years ago, the only change that kept amazing you

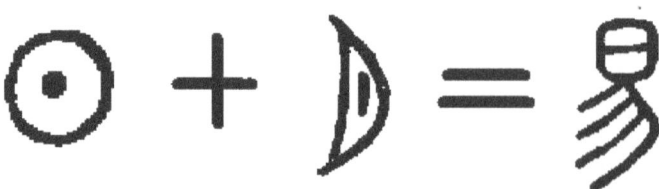

Fig. 1.2. Yi (易) in ancient Chinese form.

and yet gave you a sense of reliability was the predictable rise and fall of the sun and moon. It is logical that people started from something they knew relatively well in order to build up their knowledge system to understand the rest of the world.

Taoists are acutely aware that we are in a fast-changing world, partly due to our own activities. In order to survive in this world, we need to react properly according to the situations. To react properly, we need to have a peaceful mind in the midst of utmost chaos. This is the true reason early Taoists had for advocating *xu* (虚 empty) and *jing* (静 quiet).

This type of "empty" and "quiet" status was actually the secret of ultimate strength and power. However, in later years, this concept was gradually misinterpreted as advocating meaningless and physical weakness. In the Jin (晋) Dynasty, it even led to pervasive decadent sentiments and finally changed Chinese scholars into the least physically capable species on this planet. This tells us how dangerous it is to be a careless learner.

In a fast-changing world, it is not enough to react fast. Taoism theories try to explore the reason behind the changes and use what we have learned to guide our actions proactively.

Taoism concludes that the driver of all change is the interaction between everything and their exact opposites — 反者道之动. For example, what brings light is darkness, what brings hardness is softness, and so on. This is again *Yin* and *Yang*, which acts as the driver of all changes. No wonder *Yin* and *Yang* has become the most important concept in *Feng Shui* (风 wind 水 water), a Chinese geomantic belief that people's fortunes can be changed by changing the environment that surrounds them.

Bagua is the more refined development of *Yin* and *Yang* (Figs. 1.3 and 1.4).

It is worth noting that the "- -" here does not stand for two bars. The focus is on what is missing in between the two bars. In other words, it is the gap between the bars that matters. It is like a one-dimensional 0. The hollow part is the true meaning of the symbol.

Like the Greeks, the Chinese also found mathematics an indispensable tool to understanding the world with any accuracy. In about 500 B.C., Pythagoras was trying to make mathematics the central principle of life. It was said in about 5000 B.C., a Chinese called *Fu Xi* (伏羲)created the Bagua and tried to use it to explain everything around us in a mathematical way.

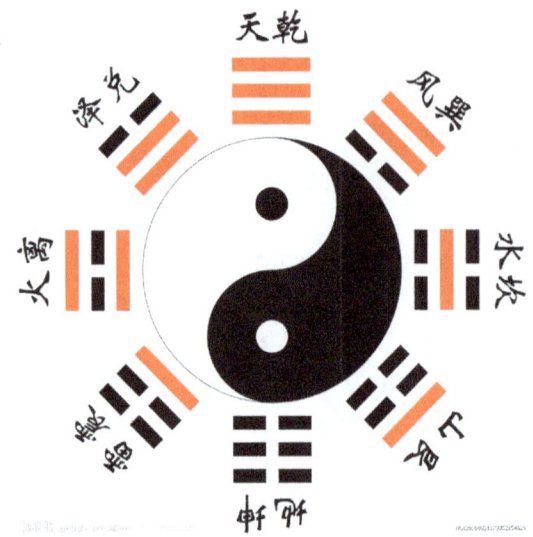

Fig. 1.3. The typical Bagua layout we see today.

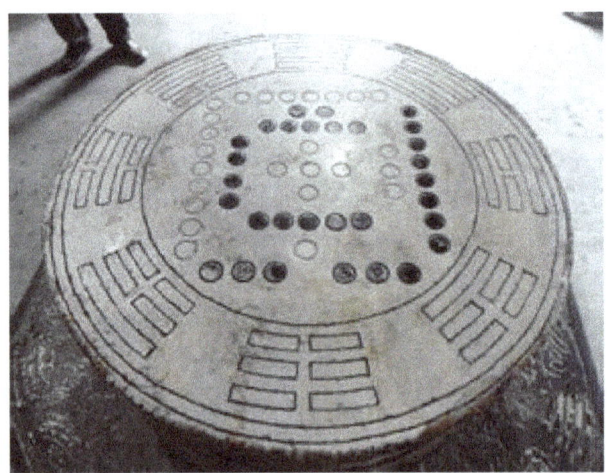

Fig. 1.4. The older Bagua layout.

On the surface, the mathematical side of Taoism still treats numbers as a container rather than the real logic behind everything. It is like the ancient people who tied knots to remember things, or modern salesmen who use bullet point listings in a presentation. However, there is something deeper than that in the narratives after each trigram.

Thousands of books have been written about the mysteriously profound *I Ching* or *Book of Changes*. However, it is not the task of this book to explain in detail the narratives and interpretations of the 64 hexagrams.

Here is the summary: the world was created originally from one *Tao*. It split into *Yin* and *Yang*, while *Yin* includes *Yang* and inside *Yang*, there is *Yin*. One more split brings us the *Si Xiang* (四 four 象 patterns). Then we have the final split from *Si Xiang* which brings us to the topic of the book: *Bagua* (八 eight 卦 Trigrams).

This coincides with the first sentence of Chapter 42 from the 《道德经》*Tao Te Ching* or *Bible of Tao* by Lao Zi: The Tao produced One; One produced Two; Two produced Three; Three produced everything else.

After the third split, there are no more splits. These eight basic combinations of three whole or broken lines form the basic set of "trigrams" to explain more complicated phenomenon. Fu Xi （伏羲） applied the combination method of mathematics and developed 64 hexagrams with all the possible combination of any two trigrams. In later years, many used these 64 trigrams in divination, leveraging on the ambiguous interpretations of the trigrams.

As the Bagua Palm is named after the eight basic trigrams, we explore it here in more detail:

☰ *Qian* (乾 heaven)

The ancient Chinese believed that heaven consists of the purest *Qi*. *Qi* is the father of all changes with positive energy and stands for an attitude of being on top of everything. That is why the emperor's residence was named *Qian* (乾 heaven) *Qing* (清 clear) *Gong* (宫 palace).

In reference to our body, *Qian* is the head.

☷ *Kun* (坤 earth)

The earth is a motherly figure in China. It is tranquil, supportive, and abundant. On top of it, everything grows. So the Queen's residence is beautifully called *Kun* (坤 earth) *Ning* (宁 peace) *Gong* (宫 palace).

In reference to our body, *Kun* is the abdomen.

☵ *Kan* (坎 water)

From the outside, water looks soft and weak. However, dripping water has the power to penetrate stone. That is the real property of water as the trigram shows, a solid core surrounded by a hollow external.

In reference to our body, *Kan* is the ear.

☲ Li (离 fire)

Fire is the opposite of water. It has a powerful edge that destroys everything, but a soft core which is not even as hot as the rim.

In reference to our body, *Li* is the heart.

☳ Zhen (震 thunder)

Thunder is almost invisible from the sky where it comes from. Only when it hits the ground does it make a big bang — a solid impact.

In reference to our body, *Zhen* is the feet.

☴ Xun (巽 wind)

Wind is the opposite of thunder. It is very visible from the sky, where it drives the clouds to shift and swirl into exotic shapes. But on the ground, we barely feel the breeze.

In reference to our body, *Xun* is the thighs.

☶ Gen (艮 mountain)

Under the hard rocky shell of the mountain, there are usually holes with gas and water.

In reference to our body, *Gen* is the hands.

☱ Dui (兑 marsh)

The trigram of the marsh is easily understandable: indicating shallow mud on top and a solid ground underneath.

In reference to our body, *Dui* is the mouth.

This set of trigrams and hexagrams and all the notes attached may look complicated and seem to go nowhere. In fact, the opposite is true. They all come from one idea: the simple and yet profound Taoism belief that everything in this world comes from one *Tao*.

There is a well-known Taoism maxim: 道法自然, which literally means that the Tao comes from nature. The trigrams and hexagrams do not come from one or two brilliant minds. They come from the inspiration of nature. As we are the children of nature, it naturally helps to know our parents in order to know ourselves better.

This simple but powerful belief has another implication: since the way of everything on earth comes from one nature, the *Tao* of every trade is similar. That means if we learn any one of the trades, say martial arts, really well, we shall find ourselves better at everything else we do. The reverse is true: if learning martial arts does not make us a better driver, we have not really learned anything.

4. The Taoists respect lives and believe in being soft.

Taoism is strong at philosophy but weak in ethics. Ethically, the most significant preaching of the Taoism is the respect of lives, which is called *hao* (好love) *sheng* (生live). They claim that nature loves lives. (天heaven 有has好love生live之's德property) This again comes from the observation in nature where the *Qi* from the heaven and earth interacts and grows everything.

As a consequence, the biggest difference of a Taoism ritual from that of all other religions is that the Taoists never kill an animal in any circumstances. All lives are honorable from the Taoism perspective. This partly explains why the Chinese in general are a giant group of very peaceful people. You do not want to imagine what might happen if one-fifth of the people on earth suddenly become aggressive or even turn savage.

The word *sheng* (生 live) also means being alive. The teachings and practices of Taoism are aimed at making people more alive. To do that, the Taoists focus on being "soft." Taoists intuitively understand the essence of live creatures. They often quote that the living weeds are soft, while the dead weeds are dry and stiff (Figs. 1.5 and 1.6).

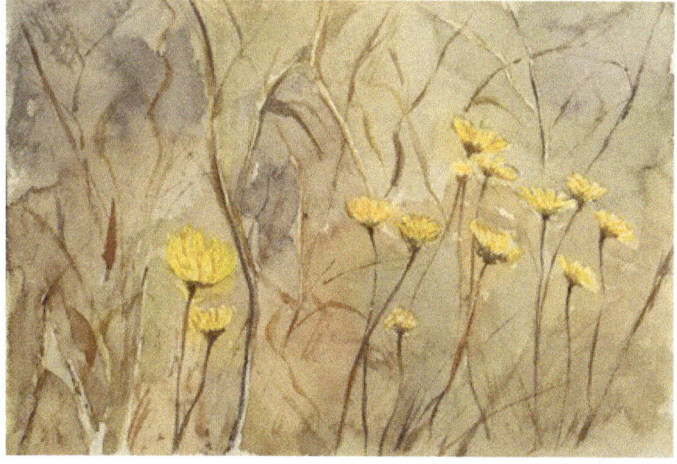

Fig. 1.5. Picture of dead weeds.

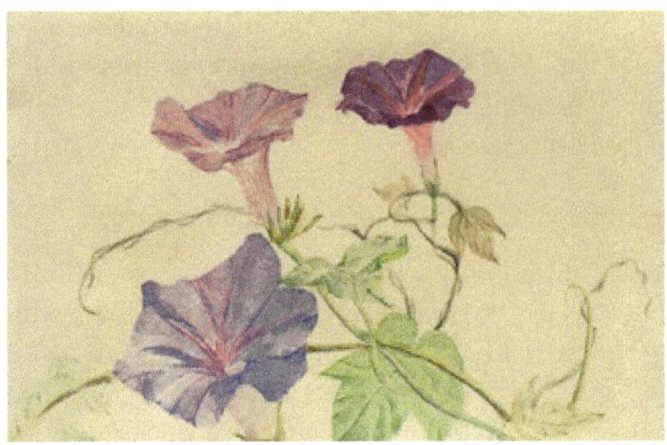

Fig. 1.6. Picture of live weeds.

From here comes the most well-known Taoism concept: the soft will always prevail. *Rou* (柔soft) *Ruo* (弱weak) *Sheng* (胜beat) *Gang* (刚hard) *Qiang* (强tough). This concept has influenced the Chinese martial arts, especially the inner school, deeply. Even the Japanese martial art Judo (柔道), also includes this concept. And the Brazilian Jujitsu, which was introduced from Japan, tells the same story with its Japanese name *Ju* (柔 soft) *Jitsu* (术 method).

There is an interesting story about a meeting between the founder of Confucianism and the founder of Taoism. One day, Confucius went to visit the aged Lao-zi, who is widely considered to be the founder of Taoism. Being old and weak, Lao-zi did not even bother to speak. He simply opened his mouth and Confucius went back in great joy of being enlightened.

Confucius's students asked him what he saw. He said: "I saw Lao-zi's tongue. It was still agile and healthy. But his teeth were all gone. He was trying to tell me that the soft is stronger than the hard." Teeth are made of hard material, but drop out the first among all our body parts.

So, this is the Taoism conclusion: soft is live; hard means dead. You will see the true meaning of this rather than the oversimplified saying in the later part of this book on Chinese martial arts.

The softest material in nature is air or *Qi* (气 gas or anything gaseous). However, this is not the reason why the Taoists want to *Qi*-lize everything. What exactly is *Qi*? It certainly is not only air, but has certain properties related to air. This might be a clue to understanding *Qi*.

First of all, air is invisible and so is *Qi*. *Qi* symbolized the ancient Chinese's understanding that the world was not only what they saw. There is something invisible which shall not be overlooked when factored into anything. Do not look at issues on the surface.

One example is, without a microscope, germs or viruses causing diseases cannot be seen. However, the Chinese did "feel" the existence of such invisible creatures and called them *Zhang* (瘴disease) *Qi*.

On the other hand, air has high mobility and changes all the time. *Qi* was thus introduced to tell people that the world around us was a changing subject and those changes might be invisible too.

The third property of air is that it is all connected as a whole. A brick has no influence on even its nearest neighbor if they do not touch each other. The liquid has limited near field influence. The air? You know the butterfly effect. Intuitively, people understand the long-range influence of the air though their observation of the weather. In this sense, nothing is better as a tool than *Qi* to be applied to explain the Taoism concept of *yin* (因cause) *guo* (果effect), especially when the cause and effect do not look very closely related.

The fact is the Taoists do use the word *Qi* often. It seems that their whole theory is built on the assumption that *Qi* is both the hot bed and death bed of everything on earth.

For example, the Taoism Gods came from *Qi*, the *Tao* (道way) itself is *Qi*, the practice of Taoism is to *zhuan* (专focus on) *Qi*, etc. The original *Qi* is called *yuan Qi* (元气) to differentiate with all other *Qi*. Those concepts are also borrowed by Chinese medicine. The *Qi* has properties such as *Yin* and *Yang*, *sheng* (盛booming) and *shuai* (衰 dying). The different types of *Qi* with different properties interact with each other and make everything happen.

As a philosophy from one of the earliest cultures in the world, Taoism pays great attention to the words and characters. It was said that when Cang (仓) Xie (颉) created the words, the heaven rained grains and the ghosts cried sadly in the evening. Actually, the Chinese word for the creation process is also one that people learn from nature. We all know that Chinese words look like simplified pictures. The words and symbols used to be the same category, and a large part of those were created by watching the pattern changes of the clouds!

Figure 1.7 shows a *Fu* (符Taoism Character), which the Taoists used to move things around.

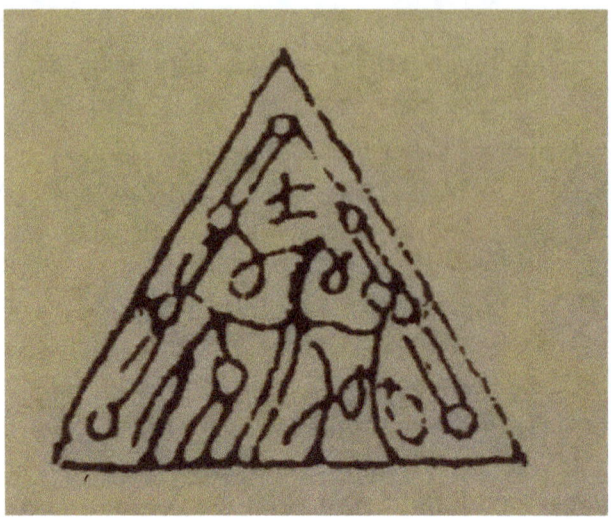

Fig. 1.7. Picture of a *Fu*.

Chinese words were made so mystic that they became sacred in some ways. People who watch Hong Kong zombie movies will find that the Taoists function like the Harry Potters of China. The difference is that they do not ride brooms or use wands and magic materials. Instead, they simply write some symbol and/or character on a piece of paper and use the power of the words to control the ghosts.

These types of tools are certainly very cost effective and versatile. However, unlike in the western world, the Taoists of ancient China had never played a major role as the keepers of the words. This role went to the Confucians, who were dominant in the preservation and creation of most written materials.

Staying in the Middle of the Road: A Chinese Attitude of Facing the Unknown

Confucianism has unquestionably been the dominant school of thought in China in recent centuries. Some younger students of Confucianism are often surprised by the simple and easy teachings, and they wonder how such teachings can be so dominant even in China, where people love simplicity.

Confucianism was created at about the same time as Taoism. It was a time of great turmoil, and people, not just the rulers, were eager for solutions. As we will analyze later, nature itself does not change that much. Physically, even human beings do not change much. What changes and keeps on changing is what comes from people's minds, the technology, the society and so on. And the speed of change is forever accelerating.

Confucianism tried to find a solution to calm people down by claiming that 天(heaven)不(does not)变(change); 道(Tao)也(also)不(does not)变(change). This claim is not absurd. Except that we keep on finding new rules, there is no evidence so far that the actual rules governing the world we know ever change. This claim is very dear to the heart of the rulers, especially the Chinese emperors, who always strove to maintain their power and pass it on peacefully, generation after generation, to their sons.

This is one of the biggest reasons why Confucianism became dominant — a powerful thought connects with power itself. And there is more.

Confucianism is a miracle compared with many famous philosophy schools from the west. It is accepted and absorbed by both the elites and the masses.

It looks simple even to beginners, so it is very suitable for people are too busy working or enjoying life to think deeply. At the same time, it can be very profound for the more aged and experienced.

It advocates universal love, extending from family members to all people in the world, but also, it has plenty of real-world advice on how to manipulate everything, which makes it appealing to both decent people and those who try to control the world in a hawkish manner.

According to *Da Xue* 《大学》, a Confucianism classic which set the targets for all beginning scholars, the ranking of lifetime achievements is as follows (from top to bottom): Resume yourself and "world peace," rule your kingdom, unite your family, improve yourself, rectify your mind, be honest and determined, get knowledge, do what you do, and observe the world. This long chain of reverse engineering is almost modern western methodology: it looks simple from each step, but makes a big achievement when combined. The approach is a very scientific and no-nonsense one.

The Confucian methodology is at once simple and complete. It all goes to believing your own original heart. We face frustration and struggle our entire lives fighting for everything and interacting with the complicated and forever changing external world only to rediscover our original heart. Some people may think simple meditation can achieve all this. Frankly speaking, I do not think so. You have to do (i.e. fighting and interacting with the external world and meditating).

The "original heart" is considered the best weapon and end result of the fight. You still need to take a right position in a real fight. This position is in the middle.

The doctrine of the mean or the golden mean (of the Confucian school) is such an important concept that one whole book out of the four books or *Si* (四four) *Shu* (书book) is dedicated to this topic.

The essence of Confucianism is to stay in the middle. It has been passed down to the most devout Confucian believers as a *Xin* (心heart) *Fa* (法method), which literally means the "core principle" that only the best of the best have the right to access. If you have watched the movie *Kungfu Panda*, you will know what it is. Yes, that was the final piece of advice which the Dragon Warrior was supposed to find in the scroll that only he was entitled to open.

The doctrine of the mean has been taught with such authority that nobody seems bothered to question why we should take such a position. There are so many positions, left and right, front and back, up and down; why should we stay in the middle? This fundamental question may leave many scholars scratching their heads, but it is actually very easy for a Chinese martial artist to answer.

In a real fight, when facing a very skilled opponent, it is very dangerous to take any position. If you lean too much to the left, you will be attacked from the left. As your muscles are already largely stretched due to the tilted position, your reaction to the attack will be limited. The same will happen if you lean too much to the right.

Only when you are in the upright middle position are your muscles in the most relaxed state, as your spine is straight and the vertebrae can stay where they are supposed to be without much help from the muscles.

At the same time, when in the middle, you are not too far from any position. This enables you to react properly with the best efficiency, especially when you have no clue what is going to happen next. Thus, staying in the middle becomes the best strategy in a chaotic world full of uncertainty.

Staying in the middle makes great sense in martial art, not only because it is the best way to handle an unpredictable change. From the angle of your opponent, by staying in the middle, you give no clue as to where you are going, so he cannot take advantage by leveraging on your intended movements.

From either side, the answer is clear. Why do you want to stay in the middle? Because you do not have a clue and you do not want to give any clues either. Thus, staying in the middle is the best strategy to face the unknown present and ever-changing future.

The Chinese are so infatuated with the middle position that they call their country *Zhong* (中 Middle) Guo (国 Kingdom), and themselves, people of the Middle Kingdom.

People outside of China sometimes have the feeling that the Chinese might be self-centric by calling their country the Middle Kingdom. Actually the "middle" here is more a philosophical positioning than a self-important type of arrogance.

People who have any real personal interaction with the Chinese will find that they are mostly modest people, or at least they try very hard to pretend to be so. So the "middle" here is more about a way they carry themselves. They do not want to be too much in any direction. This explains why there have been so few extremists in China in Chinese history.

Such a simple posture can best prepare you to handle the worst disasters to come in many cases. However, any rules are subject to situations. It would lead to absolute disaster if anyone follows a rule with a rigid mind. For example, if you are walking in the street, walking in the middle of the street is not safe.

Perhaps it is well to remember that we are talking about just the martial arts while trying to justify the middle-of-the-road position. However, staying in the middle might be a good option in helping us to understand situations when we do not know what will happen. (In this book on martial arts, we have devoted this entire first chapter to Chinese culture. And in this chapter about Chinese culture, we have just discussed the martial arts for a whole page. This is called "*Yin* inside *Yang* and *Yang* inside *Yin*" as Fig. 1.8 shows.)

As illustrated by the *Yin Yang* Fish, in real situations, there is always some opposite ingredient or factor inside everything. Nothing is pure. This is another discourse about the doctrine of the mean.

Unlike the impression of many people, the mysterious *Book of Changes* 《易经》 is not only a Taoism bible. It is also one of the classics

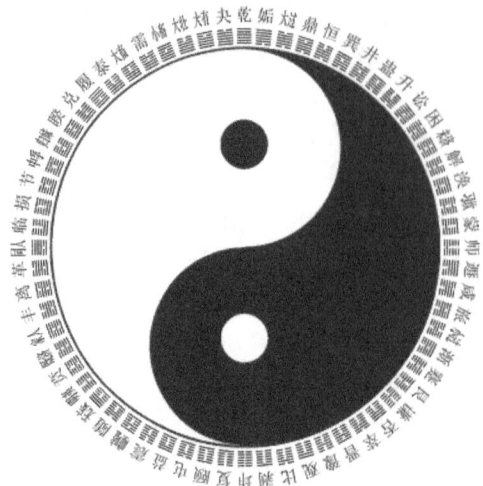

Fig. 1.8. *Yin Yang* Fish.

of Confucianism. When Fu Xi developed the 64 hexagrams, there were no explanations, and Confucius himself finished that job.

The *Book of Changes* was Confucius's favorite book. He read it so often that the binding of the book broke many times. If you read his words of explanation through 《论语》, you will find them very vivid and alive, full of surprises and changing points according to situations and contexts.

However, not all the students of Confucius were as talented as Confucius. In the Han Dynasty, as Confucianism became officially dominant in China, many of his doctrines became rigid rules.

When Confucius said, "The nature does not change and neither does the Tao," he was trying to say the rules behind what was going on, such as the law of nature remained the same. This should give us the confidence that we can learn from the previous wise people to understand the world better. However, this was interpreted by many as a command that we should never do anything to change the world, as it is futile to do so.

As Confucianism's basic edict is to stay in the middle of the road, it gives many mediocre and lazy people the perfect excuse not to move forward to explore the unknown. Fortunately, the Chinese had Taoism, which advocated change, as the second dominant culture. Even so, the Chinese had a really hard time in the recent 200 years due to their conservative culture.

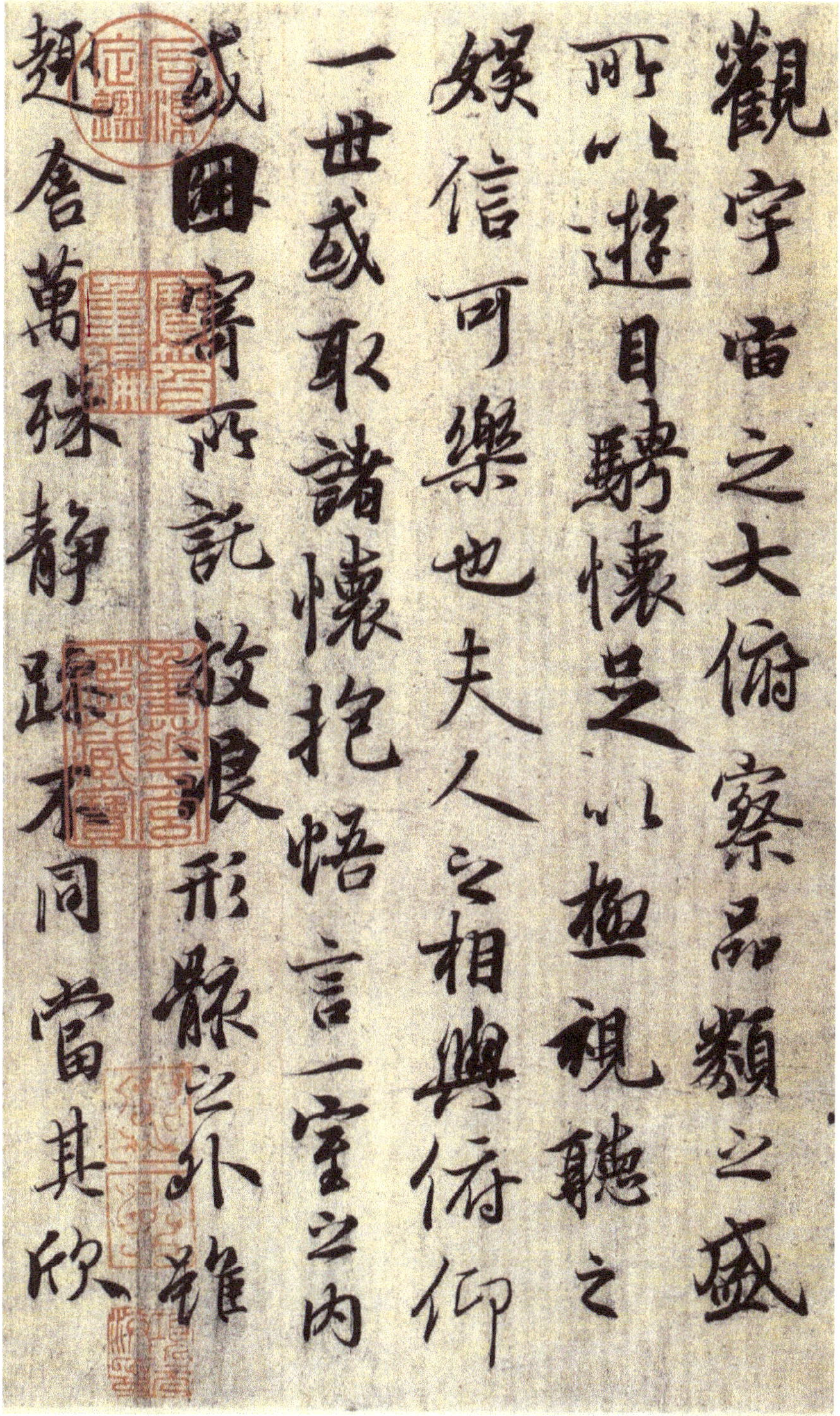

観宇宙之大俯察品類之盛所以遊目騁懷足以極視聽之娛信可樂也夫人之相與俯仰一世或取諸懷抱悟言一室之內或因寄所託放浪形骸之外雖趣舍萬殊靜躁不同當其欣

Fig. 1.9. *Lan Ting Xu* (兰亭序).

On the other hand, with all the negatives in the culture for over 2000 years, especially after the recent 200 miserable years, the Chinese has still remained the biggest population on this planet. You have to be amazed about the great vitality in Chinese culture, which is not dying yet. It is merging with other cultures and will surely contribute positively to a better future.

We can summarize this chapter with a small example. In typical Chinese funerals, the most frequently told words are 节哀顺变 — Be prudent in sorrow and go with the changes. This is to console people who have lost their family members. Even while people feel sad, they should not go to extremes, as their energy should be saved to handle all the changes to come. This short sentence combines the two most popular concepts from Confucianism and Taoism — to stay in the middle and be prepared for the changes.

People do not talk nonsense in funerals. So, let us remember the key points here: Stay in the middle and be prepared for the changes.

Lan Ting Xu (兰亭序), the highest standard of Chinese calligraphy, shows both great stability and capability to change (Fig. 1.9).

We will see a lot of applications of these two concepts in the chapters to come.

2
Further Development of Chinese Martial Arts

The Chinese kept good historical records. Each dynasty since the Xia Dynasty (about 4000 years ago), would assign officers dedicated to recording and keeping history.

Some neighboring countries even used the ancient Chinese recordings as the only reliable ancient history that existed, such as Cambodia during the Angkor Dynasty. A great part of ancient Indian history would not be complete without the Chinese files, which were written by the Chinese Buddhists who traveled to India to learn Buddhism.

However, there was almost nothing recorded about Chinese martial arts in the official histories. A 2000-year-old fairy tale briefly described the sword skills of a young lady named *Yue Nu*, whose skills were taught by a white monkey (Fig. 2.1). That gives us a clue as to why there are so many Chinese martial art postures named after animals, especially monkeys.

The only related things officially recorded were the deeds of the generals. This reflects Chinese achievement-oriented values: it is not about what you can do, much less about what you could have done, but all about what you have done. Succeed, and you are the king; lose, and you are a mere bandit — 成 (succeed) 王 (king) 败 (lose) 寇 (bandit).

The early records on martial arts were all about weapons skills, from the sword play of Lady *Yue Nu* to General *Li Guang* of the Han Dynasty, who was famous for his archery skills. General Li once shot an arrow deep into a stone even when he was drunk. He earned his nickname, Flying General, from a fight where he was heavily wounded and captured by the Hun army. Magically, he managed to jump over and in between the two

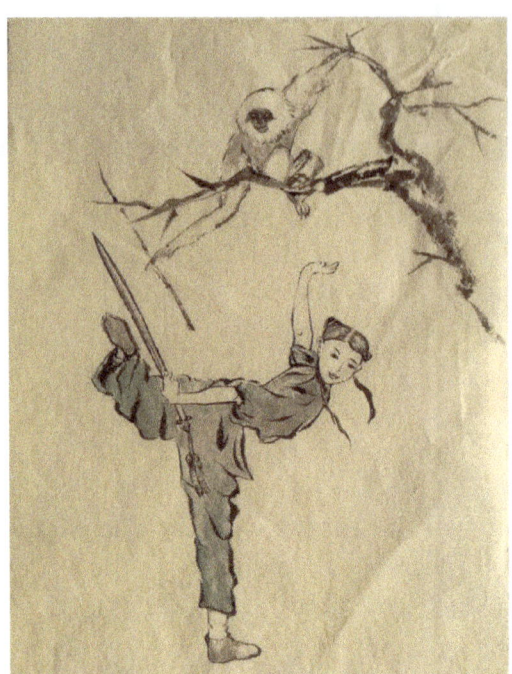

Fig. 2.1. The sword of *Yue Nu*.

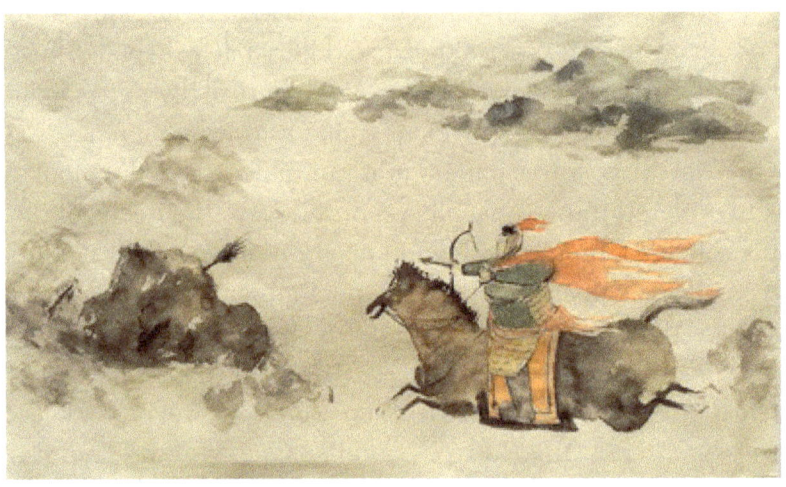

Fig. 2.2. "Flying General" *Li Guang*.

horses carrying him and kill a Hun soldier, grab his bow and horse, and shoot all his enemies, finally rejoining his own army.

The highest ranked Chinese martial artist was the first emperor of the Song Dynasty, Zhao Kuang Yin. He was famous for his bludgeoning skills and even more famous for protecting a young lady and traveling a thousand miles to send her home. It is worth noting that the young lady was a stranger to him, and he had never even touched her in the process or after that. Zhao led a life like a Chinese version of King Arthur, except he was not the son of a king but was "made" emperor by the generals who followed him.

As a great martial artist, Zhao certainly knew what martial art could do. He disarmed all the generals who supported him and redesigned the whole government system, channeling all the power into the hands of non-military officials. At the same time, weapon play was not encouraged and the focus of Chinese martial arts became more *Kong* (空 empty) *Shou* (手 hand) style, which the Japanese now called Karate.

As the body tires easily, it is not able to sustain a long drawn-out fight with weapons. The non-weapon type of martial art is more technique oriented, and fought one-on-one. In time, martial arts became practiced more for self-cultivation than for actual killing.

There are generally two big schools of Chinese martial arts: the outer school and the inner school. The outer school is mostly very fierce when practicing, and the most famous big clan is called Shaolin — named after the Buddhist temple famous for being the birth place of the Chinese Zen clan. The inner school, on the other hand, is normally practiced at a much slower pace. The most famous clan here is Wudang, named after a Taoist temple.

All Martial Arts Come from Shaolin — 天下武功出少林

People usually believe that the outer school is designed more for fighting and the inner school, such as the famous *Tai Chi* (太 grand 极 utmost), is mostly for wellness purposes. Ironically, the stories about the origin of those martial arts point to almost the opposite.

The weapon used in practice by the Muslin Chinese martial artist Wang Zi Ping is called Bodhi dharma's spade. Wang Zi Ping used to be the Chief of the Shaolin Clan in the Central Institute of Chinese Martial Arts.

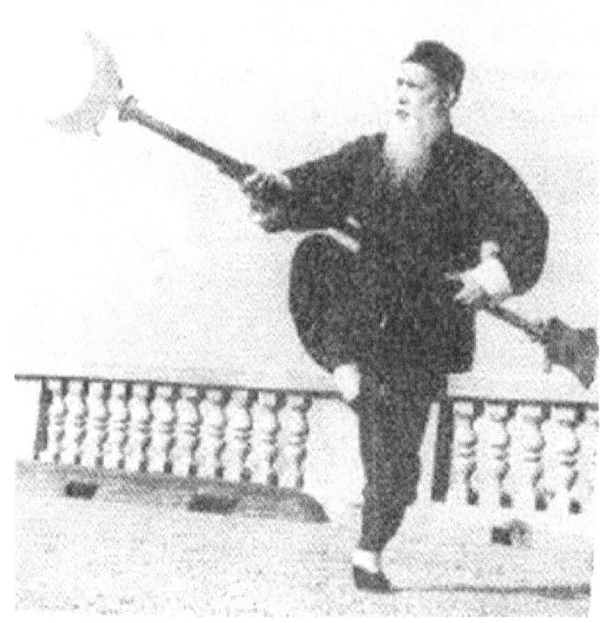

Fig. 2.3. Wang Zi Ping practicing with Bodhi dharma's spade.

It is widely believed that the Shaolin, as the original Zen clan in China, was built by an Indian monk — Bodhi dharma or *da* (达 reach) *mo* (摩 touch) in Chinese. Bodhi dharma was a master of Zen, which later became the most influential branch of Buddhism in northeast Asia. He found that his students were physically weak due to sitting all day and meditating without any exercise. He then created some forms of exercises to strengthen his students. Those exercises became the foundation of Shaolin martial arts. So initially, Shaolin martial art was not created for fighting, but for the wellness of the Zen students. Of course it did not stop there, or it would not have become the Shao Lin martial art as we know it today.

Fighting was not an art in China until different kinds of fighting skills were introduced into the famous Shaolin Temple, where they were merged and reorganized into a giant system of martial arts.

It takes great consistency to fine-tune an art, generation after generation. The Shaolin Temple, with its fame in martial arts society and 1500 years of patriarchal clan-style management, provided that consistency.[1] That is why there is a saying that all the martial arts in the "world" (which means China), comes from Shao Lin — 天下武功出少林.

The Shaolin Temple was not built in one day. Neither was the Shaolin clan of martial arts. It includes so many systems and styles that no one can ever imagine himself learning everything there is to learn about Shaolin even if he studied it his entire life.

People tend to regard all the outer-school Chinese martial arts as Shaolin. However, the real Shaolin is much more rigorous in style and methodology. Influenced by Zen philosophy, the Shaolin style is extremely straightforward with no unnecessary movements. There are no far-reaching large-scales movements. The punch and defense are through short paths. It is advocated that the Shaolin Gongfu can be practiced in any place big enough for an ox to lie down.

It is not a coincidence that Shaolin as a Zen temple was regarded as the center for all outer-school Chinese martial art. The Zen which Bodhi dharma passed to the Chinese includes a whole set of elements that is crucial for the success of a martial artist: the ruthless self-torturing physical challenge, the separation from the temptations of normal life, and the search for clarity of the mind and spirit through self-enlightenment.

Actually, Shaolin as a clan or a temple is more a spiritual symbol than a physical body. Due to its ultimate position is Chinese martial arts, it attracts the masters from all over China to study and exchange their skills in and out of the temple. All those activities not only strengthened the position of Shaolin as a Chinese martial arts emblem, but also gave birth to the inner style of martial arts, which at first glance is very different from Shaolin.

The Evolution from Outer School to Inner School

Unlike the outer school, the core of the inner school of martial arts is not the thousands of forms from numerous clans. The core of the inner school of martial arts is invisible; it is a set of principles and rules stemming from those principles. The principles are largely coherent with the Taoism teachings, and thus the inner school is in many cases treated equal to the Wudang (a Taoist temple) clan.

Compared with the outer school, the inner school is relatively new and much more consolidated. The biggest clans are the famous Xingyi, Tai Chi, and Bagua.

Xingyi is the earliest clan of the inner school and is well known for its explosive power. Its core form is called *wu* (五 five) *xing* (行 elements) *quan* (拳 fist), which has five forms connected to the five elements theory of Chinese philosophy. The five forms are so simple that you can finish learning them in five minutes. However, many people may spend their entire lives practicing and still not get even one form right without a decent teacher. The countless changes in the different *jing* (勁 force) of the five forms make Xingyi one of the toughest martial arts to learn as well as the most used martial art technique applied in the real battlefield.

From the way Master Sun Lu Tang sits, we can learn a lot about the inner school of Chinese Martial Arts (Fig. 2.4). He sits up straight and yet

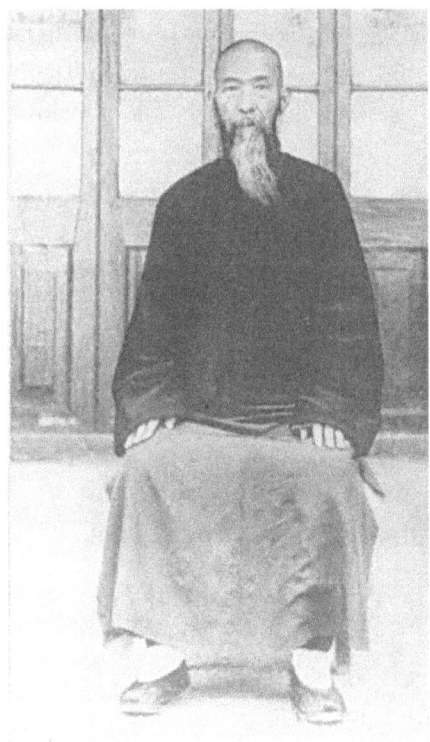

Fig. 2.4. Master Sun Lu Tang.

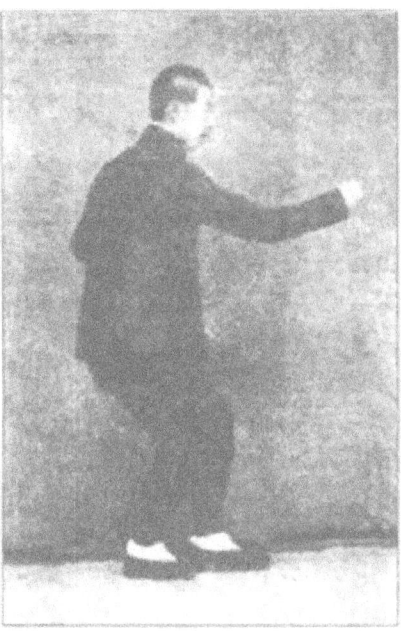

Fig. 2.5. Half-step bursting fist.

is relaxed (look at his shoulders), gazing peacefully and horizontally, palms flexed. This is not a new picture. I saw it many times many years ago. But it is only recently when I started to understand why he is the best of the best, just from looking at the picture. There is something there that is difficult to qualify, let alone quantify, even for a trained physicist — his Qi.

The typical Xingyi is best demonstrated by one of its masters, Guo Yun Shen, who set the foundation for what Xingyi looks like nowadays. Instead of applying different techniques from the complicated Chinese martial arts system, he is famous for using his unique "half-step bursting fist" to defeat all martial artists who dared to challenge him. The full name for this technique is 半(half)步(step)崩(bursting)拳(fist)打(beat)天下(the world).

He even told his opponents what he would do before the fight. Everyone knew what was coming, but still could not handle it when they saw it. Just one stroke, not even the five forms, in the simplest way! That is the essence of the inner-style martial arts: the yi (意 mind) is much more important than the $xing$ (形 form).

To better illustrate the importance of the yi (意 mind), let us examine how master Guo's unique "half-step bursting fist" was developed. It happened when Guo was chained in jail as a felon after he killed a bad guy. Because the chains were too short, Guo could not even complete one full step when he tried to practice the "bursting fist." His solution was to shorten his step to half the length of his normal step. Thus, the unique "half-step bursting fist" was formed.

In Chinese martial arts, being accurate is quite important in practicing. Such changes are not allowed normally. Especially for this form, which was developed over generations, such change may even make it ineffective.

Those who tried to explain Guo's success in perfecting his "half-step bursting fist" normally attributed it to his hardworking spirit even when he was in jail. That is certainly part of it, but not even the most important part of it, much less all of it.

Being deprived of his freedom when he was in the jail actually gave Guo a unique advantage — focus. That environment of ultimate deprivation granted Guo extreme focus when he was practicing. There were no friends, no foes. As a chained felon in that small cell, he did not have a hope, which meant he did not even have much of himself to think about.

Nothing ever bothered him because, after all, there was nothing. The only thing left was martial arts, and perhaps the shackles. He entered a state similar to an experienced monk in meditation. That kind of intensive focus enlightened Guo and allowed him to master his *yi* (意 mind) and finally join his *yi* and *xing* (形 body) into one. That is the true source of his massive power displayed in his unique "half-step bursting fist."

The muscles built through hard work can degenerate. The swiftness of skill obtained through intensive training can get rusty. The enlightenment that happens in such an extreme environment will never disappear, just like a burn mark on a tree from a great lightning strike.

The Xingyi is very similar in its forms with *Xin* (心 heart) *Yi* (意 mind) — a famous Shaolin form, while Taiji looks like a totally different type of martial art in many ways.

However, as many other martial arts, Taiji also has its sources connected to Shaolin. Based on many people's belief, the whole inner school of martial arts, including Taiji, was initialed by a Taoist called Zhang San Feng. A famous scholar, Huang Zong Xi, noted that Zhang San Feng, who used to be very good at Shaolin, redesigned the forms and rules and created the inner school of martial arts.[2] Who the actual original creator of Taiji is, is a highly controversial topic. However, there is little argument about where the Taiji we are practicing now comes from. It all came from a brilliant young genius called Yang Lu Chan who learned the art from a small village called Chen Jia Gou and brought it to Beijing, the capital city of the Qing Dynasty.

Beijing was the biggest platform for any martial artist then to make a name for himself. The city had never heard of anything like Taiji before Yang. In Beijing, where all the best of the best martial artists stayed, Yang fought with all the challengers and never lost a single fight. Thus, he got the nickname Matchless Yang.

As he became the most famous martial artist in Beijing, many people from the royal family followed him to learn Taiji. Those were simply not the strongest people and found Taiji tough to learn. So Yang modified the original Taiji and made it easier for ordinary people to practice. Today Taiji has become the most practiced Chinese martial arts in the world with many modified versions.

Taiji is the most thorough inner-style martial art in terms of its form, principles, and the way it is practiced. It looks so slow and soft that it is hard to imagine anyone fighting with such skills. However, Yang Lu Chan himself was the best example, showcasing the power of this "soft" martial arts style. Yang was of a relatively small build. All his opponents were much stronger and bigger, and yet all lost to him. The way he handled his opponents was also very impressive. He moved extremely fast, and was as agile as a monkey, and his hands always moved in a circular way as if he was holding a ball. This was definitely something people had never seen then.

One of the most famous scholars, Wen Tong He, was so impressed after observing Yang's Taiji that he praised the style "as all rounded and complete as a Tai Ji." This is the origin of the official name of Taiji Quan.

The actual core of Taiji is a set of principles. Following that set of principles, one can easily practice any other style of Chinese martial art and make it look exactly like Taiji.

Taiji has included the most complete, modern, and scientific martial art principles. However, what really sets Taiji apart is not the principles but rather the way it has spread all over the world.

Taiji was the first Chinese martial art that was opened to the public. Before Yang Lu Chan, Taiji was only taught to family members in a small village called Chen Jia Gou, where almost all families in the village belong to the Chen Clan. Even in that village, Taiji was seldom taught from one family to another. Only very few families had a relatively good grasp of this art. Luckily, Yang's Taiji master was from the family that had the best knowledge of Taiji.

The same was true for all other martial arts clans. The martial art skills were usually only passed to the students in a one-to-one style. The great Gongfu masters were extremely careful about choosing their disciples. They did not want to teach those less talented so as not to embarrass themselves by having their disciples defeated by those of the other schools. Also, those who were emotionally unstable or had ethical issues had no chance to be picked. The last thing the masters wanted was to spend their life time teaching only to create trouble for themselves. Many of the masters ended up not having even one disciple until their last day on earth.

The situation in Beijing was quite different from the village Chen Jia Gou. Those who followed Yang Lu Chan to study Taiji were mostly privileged people in society, such as the royal family members and high-ranking officers and their family members.

They were not the traditional disciples who followed the old-time masters. The fundamental difference was that they were intellectuals. The intellectuals in China followed totally different rules in studying and teaching. While in martial arts most secrets were then kept in the great masters' minds, there were never any artificially kept secrets in Confucianism. Every single key point was written down on paper, black and white, in the limited number of classics. The only bottleneck for all students was their ability to understand and apply what they had learned.

As the students in Beijing were not only literate but also of even higher social status than the masters, they broke all the rules by not only exchanging what they learned among themselves but also publicly teaching other people as they wished. This caused the explosive spread of Taiji, and partly because of the first-runner effect (just like Google as a search engine and Facebook in social media today), Taiji became the most practiced Chinese martial arts in the world.

With its magnificent theory system, and great effectiveness in both fighting and self-cultivating, together with the massive market share among the martial artists, it would be very reasonable to expect Taiji to be the last revolutionary new school of martial arts. This was almost true, except that Bagua Zhang, which started to spread less than 200 years ago, was even newer, and at least equally powerful and sophisticated.

The Development of Bagua Palm As the Newest Traditional Chinese Martial Art

Bagua Palm was introduced by Master Dong Hai Chuan (Fig. 2.6) in the late Qing Dynasty, the latest in history among all the traditional Chinese martial arts. Ironically, it was the only one without a history, at least among the four most famous types of martial arts dominating Beijing in late Qing Dynasty, namely Taiji, Xingyi, Bagua and Pao Chui from the Three Emperors.

Master Dong himself also emerged as a master with a very vague history: all that people knew about him was that he was born in Wen'an County of Hebei Province as a farmer, who had been trained by Taoists in An Hui province and stayed in Shaolin temple for a few years studying martial arts.[3]

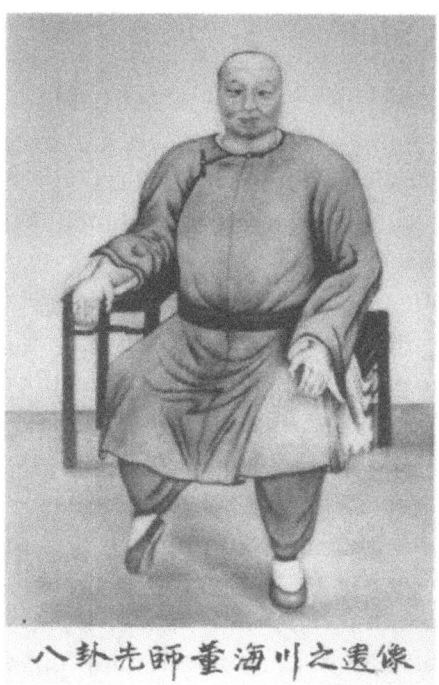

Fig. 2.6. Master Dong Hai Chuan.

Even though it is clear that Master Dong Hai Chuan introduced Bagua Palm in around 1865, it is not clear as to whether Bagua Palm was actually invented by Master Dong or was passed to him by a few Taoists.

Bagua Palm is such a peculiar Chinese martial art that it is hard to find clues from any other martial art forms. This again was not the case for any other Chinese martial art forms. For example, in Taiji we can find many forms which are very similar to Pao Chui, which is a very old Chinese martial art. A large volume of the Taiji theories was also copied from Xingyi, which entered the public world much earlier.

Xingyi itself is no exception. A large part of its famous Twelve Animal Forms are very similar to the Xin Yi's Ten Animal Forms. And Xin Yi is part of Shaolin.

When Bagua Palm appeared in Beijing, the martial art society then was astonished not just because of master Dong's effortless defeat of all the challengers, but also because of the form's countless dazzling circular footwork and spiral body and arm movements. It looked like something from another planet!

Most of the previous martial arts focused on taking a solid stance and hitting hard as hard can be. Even today, some old-school Chinese martial artists would watch the boxing steps and cannot help being amused, because they think there is too much jumping around in the footwork.

There are some schools of Chinese martial arts with swift footwork and fast hands. Cuo Jiao Fan Zi and Pi Gua are among the most famous. However, Bagua is totally different from Cuo Jiao Fan Zi in that the latter focuses on attacking with legs and it does not include any spiraling of arms and body movements.

Bagua is also different from Pi Gua, a northern Chinese martial art form, which enables the masters to fly like a swallow and hit like a whip. Pi Gua does undulate a lot but does not have that many turns and is nowhere near circular in its footwork. Pi Gua also has a lot of jumping, while in Bagua, just as in all other inner-school martial arts, you do not see any jumping at all.

It is hard enough to be different: the chances may be one in a hundred. It is much harder to win all the time without a scratch, the chances maybe less than one in ten thousand. Master Dong Hai Chuan managed to do both. This makes him a one-in-a-million phenomenon among the Chinese martial artists.

One of the more convincing explanations of the origin of Bagua is that it was modified from one of the very ancient Taoism exercises called *Zhuan* (转 turn) *Xian* (先 pre) *Tian* (天 heaven). It is worth noting that in Taoism, *Xian Tian*, which literally means pre-heaven, stands for what the Taoists think the state of people originally was, and to which they should try to return. Usually it is a concept used in self-cultivating practices.

Although Bagua is the youngest among the three major inner schools of Chinese martial art styles, Master Dong was significantly older when he dedicated himself to pass down the new style. That was in 1874, when, already 77 years old, he retired from his job with the royal family and started to teach Bagua full time. It was natural for him to pay more emphasis on self-cultivation rather than on pure fighting.

It has long been a critical topic for the elder Chinese martial artists to stay fit while aging. Fighting is destroying for both parties involved. Even the training can be destroying to the body if not done properly. Long-term health can even be intentionally sacrificed to gain short-term power with certain methods.

However, unlike boxing or any other sport, Chinese martial art was a lifetime career for many of the fighters involved. Even if they wanted to quit, the foes they made during their career might not allow them to. This is also partially the reason why the Chinese martial artist is so obsessed with the idea of being able to defeat the young even when he is old.

Bagua also has a more direct link to Taoism compared with Taiji and Xingyi. As longevity is almost the most important target for Taoists, it is also natural that Bagua has so many wellness ingredients weaved into it.

A typical set of Chinese martial art forms usually consists of three different groups of components according to the applications. The core part is for attacking and defending, or so-called practical fighting applications. A large part is for body-building and wellness, which includes flexibility, strength of different parts of the body, and power-releasing skills. This part confuses many beginners who think that all the movements in Chinese martial arts have fighting applications. The most controversial part is the dancing part, which is for performing or even entertaining, sometimes even with music as purely dance performances.

The fundamentalists believe the third part is something unnecessary or even poisoning. They think this part makes Chinese martial arts seem weak and impractical. Actually, the dancing was part of Chinese martial arts from day one. With this artistic ingredient, the practitioner actually achieved better understanding of the rhythm of the movements and better coordination. Bruce Lee, the most famous Chinese martial artist known in the west for his powerful punches and kicks, was even a semi-professional dancer.

As the newest form of traditional Chinese martial art, Bagua Palm is well developed in all the three parts. Master Dong himself is the best example. He defeated all challengers with ease and even grace. He showed stunning essential techniques, such as speed and power. At the same time, his performance in front of the royal family members was beyond impressive, and accomplished with great coordination and charm.

Master Dong was a complete martial artist. This enabled him to teach different people with a totally different approach. It was said that he did not even teach Bagua to all his students. Mostly, he only taught them Luo Han Fist, a basic Shaolin form. I believe it was not because he was trying to keep any secrets, but rather because he believed that Shaolin was indispensible for anyone who wanted to really grasp the spirit of Chinese martial arts.

Master Dong taught many people, but the most famous ones were those who already had very good martial art fundamentals before learning Bagua. Some of them were even already martial art masters by the time they started to follow Master Dong. We can regard them as his major disciples.

As Master Dong was such a complete master of Chinese martial arts, he interpreted martial art at a much higher level. The several disciples he hand-picked were from totally different background and their skills were at very different levels, but they all became great fighters.

This shows that Master Dong really understood what to look for in a person to pick a potential master. It also shows that Master Dong was very good at teaching as well. For a normal master, having experience in other forms of martial art was almost certainly a headache rather than an advantage, as he would have to "forget" what he had learnt and adjust back to the present form.

Unlike most other masters, Master Dong taught all his major disciples very differently from the very beginning. The difference came not just from the different physical characteristics of these disciples but also their personalities, and even from what they learnt before.

Till today, not much is known about Master Dong himself or even the type of Bagua he himself actually practiced. The Bagua we learn today came mostly from his first generation of major disciples.

The most well-known and recognized disciples of the first generation were Yin Fu (尹福), Cheng Ting Hua (程廷华), Liang Zhen Fu (梁振甫), Liu Feng Chun (刘凤春), Song Yong Nian (宋永年), Wei Ji (魏吉), Ma Wei Qi (马维祺), and Shi Ji Dong (史计栋). Among them, Yin Fu and Cheng Ting Hua were the two most influential disciples.

Yin Fu was widely recognized as Master Dong's top disciple. As Master Yin had extensive training in Luo Han Fist and Tan Kicking before he started to learn from Master Dong, his style consisted of a lot of kicking and lightning-quick power-releasing movements.

Cheng Ting Hua was a wrestler with relatively less martial arts background when he started following Master Dong. Cheng Ting Hua was also very tall with great strength, the same as Master Dong. So it is widely believed that Cheng Ting Hua's forms were the closest to that of Master Dong himself. The fact that Cheng Ting Hua taught most of the students for Master Dong enhanced his status as the most influential disciple of Bagua Palm.

Besides his fellow students in Bagua Palms, Master Cheng Ting Hua also taught three Xingyi masters Li Cun Yi (李存义), Zhang Zhan Kui

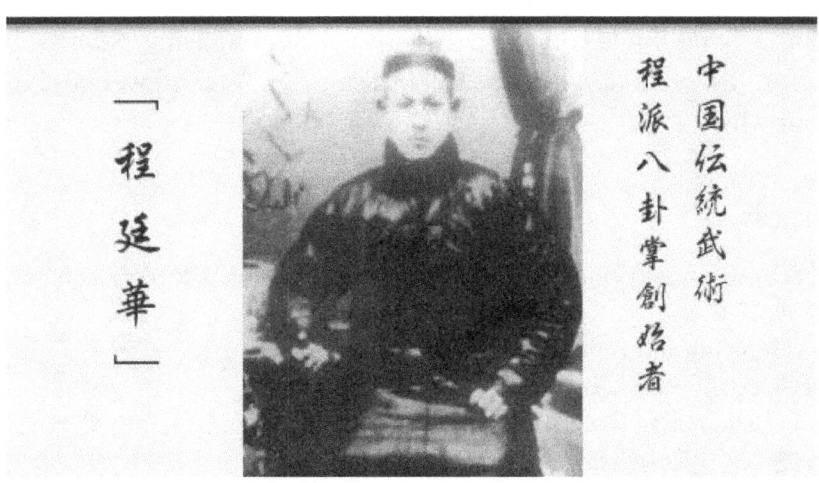

Fig. 2.7. Master Cheng Ting Hua.

(张占魁), and Liu De Kuan (刘德宽). All of them were then the top martial artists in China.

The forms introduced in this book — the Weaving Stance Bagua 64 Palms — were created by master Cheng Ting Hua.

The Bagua passed down by Master Cheng Ting Hua is now practiced by most among all the Bagua practitioners and is called Cheng Style Bagua Palms.

The Cheng Style Bagua is characterized with more twisting, circling, and spiral movements of the arms and body. It also has wider strides and bigger range in all other movements in general.

Contrary to some people's impression of Bagua Palm as a delicate martial arts, Master Cheng's performance was full of power. It gave people the impression that they were watching a giant python undulating around. That is the reason the Cheng Style Bagua also was called "Dragon Shape (龙形)" or "Continuously Linked (连环)" Bagua. The Bagua style in this book is called *You* (游 swimming) *Sheng* (身 body) Bagua which used to be literally translated as Swimming Body Bagua. Actually this *You* (游 swimming) here has nothing to do with swimming. It describes a status of being extremely agile, flexible, and unpredictable with complex undulating, twisting, and circling. The *Sheng* (身 body) here is not exactly just a body but a way of body movement. The Cheng Style Bagua moves put you in mind of someone weaving in and out between cars, where frequent changes in direction are needed to avoid the cars, thus the name "the Weaving Stance Bagua 64 Palms."

The Cheng Style Bagua, particularly the Weaving Stance Bagua 64 Palms, has great applications in both self-defense and wellness. Let us find out why.

References

1. Lu Hong Jun and Teng Lei (2012). *Shaolin Gong Fu*, p. 2, 少林功夫, 吕宏军, 滕磊, 文化艺术出版社 2012 年.
2. Lu Hong Jun and Teng Lei (2012). *Shaolin Gong Fu*, p. 155, 少林功夫, 吕宏军, 滕磊, 文化艺术出版社 2012年.
3. Wang Zhen Shan (2009). *Rou Sheng Bagua Zhang*, p. 2, 柔身八卦掌, 王振山, 人民体育出版社, 2009 年.

3
How would Sir Isaac Newton Interpret Chinese Martial Arts:
A New Scientific Approach to the Understanding of Chinese Martial Arts

Despite conventional thinking, Chinese martial arts can be explained using scientific systems rather than oriental mysticism. This chapter is devoted to the scientific interpretation of Chinese martial arts.

The beauty of classical physics has two aspects. One lies in its absolute accuracy in predicting what is going to happen by pure calculation. Before an experiment, a physicist can do a calculation and end up finding out that his calculation matches the result of the experiment practically close to 100%.

The other is the simplicity of the theory itself, which reflects a clear mind. This tradition can be traced from Einstein to Euclid. Newton's laws include only two very clear sentences and one simple formula. These explain almost all the activities of all visible objects in the known universe. I will attempt to explain Chinese martial arts using three fundamental axioms.

Axiom 1: Force Is a Vector (The Σ: Direction Matters)

The first step of scientific research is always to ask the right questions and then try to answer them.

Why is it Possible for the Weak to Defeat the Strong, The Slow to Defeat the Fast, And the Old to Defeat the Young?

Chinese martial art is obsessed with a special type of capability: the capability of being weak but able to defeat the strong, being slow but able to defeat the fast, and especially, being old but able to defeat the young.

As anti-intuitive as it is, from the point of view of Newtonian mechanics, the trick is unbelievably simple. It comes from one simple fact, that both force and velocity are vectors — quantities that not only have magnitude but also direction.

At any point in time, one force has only one direction, which means perpendicular to it, the force is zero. That is why a much smaller force can change the direction of a bigger force and lead it nowhere.

In Fig. 3.1, forces are shown as arrows. The relative length of the arrow indicates the magnitude of the force; the direction of the arrow indicates the direction of the force.

As Fig. 3.1 shows, $F1 + F2 = F$, and thus $F = F1 + F2$. Two or more forces with different directions can be combined into one force. One force can also be divided into many forces. In this case, F1 and F2 can be regarded as components of F.

If there are more than two forces, then $F = F1 + F2 + F3 \ldots$ can be expressed as $F = \Sigma Fn$. Σ stands for the combination of all components in a group.

From the division side, no matter how big the magnitude of F is, it is impossible to have a component perpendicular to F.

From the combination side, no matter how big the magnitude of F1 is, a much smaller F2 can join F1 and make the combined final force change direction.

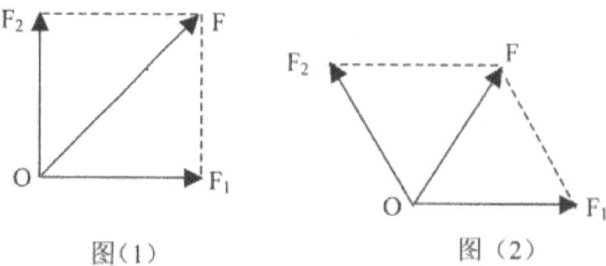

Fig. 3.1. Superposition of the forces.

This is the trick of the direction-changing game in Chinese martial arts. When the direction of the force applied by an attacker is changed, the target is safe from any damage. The attack is dissolved.

A famous Chinese martial arts saying by a Taiji master is "四两拨千斤" which literally means a force as small as 200g can change the direction of a force of 500 kg. The hint is obvious here: the word "拨" is to apply force perpendicular to the original direction and get things moving sideways.

However, in reality it is easier said than done, especially in a game with rules limiting unorthodox body contact, such as boxing. It is very hard to imagine that in the face of a trained boxer, when a jab comes your way at lightning speed, you can actually react with a perpendicular movement to block the jab effectively. By the time you see it coming, it is already too late. In real boxing, the actual trick is not to keep watching all the time and reacting. Making constant and unpredictable movements before you even know the hits are coming is the way to dodge them.

In street fights, however, irregular circling movements help, as in that case the direction and even magnitude of the speed and force change all the time, which makes it very difficult for anyone, even trained boxers, to connect and hit the target hard and accurately.

At the same time, hand blocks, which apply vertical forces relative to the attacking opponent, work just fine, as once in contact, hands can get "stickier" and the speed of the movements will be lowered dramatically, which leave great space for a weaker but smarter player to apply vertical force to change the game.

Now we go to the second question.

Why do we See so Many Circular Movements in the Practice of the Chinese Martial Arts, Especially Bagua Palm?

The Bagua form of martial art is well known for its circular movements. Again, the reason can be found easily from modern mechanics, in an elegant way.

What characterizes a round movement? When and only when the external force applied on an object is perpendicular to its velocity, will the object move in a perfect circle (Fig. 3.2).

In Fig. 3.2, the arrow F, which points to the center of the circle, is the force applied; the arrow v, which is tangential, is the velocity.

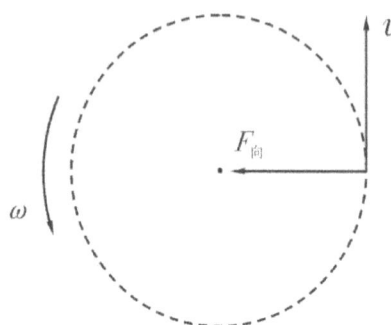

Fig. 3.2. An object moving in a perfect circle.

By definition, a tangential vector is perpendicular to the radius pointing to the center.

A small experiment can prove that whenever a uniform circular motion is observed, F must be perpendicular to v.

When we fix a small stone to one end of a rope and roll it, we see a perfect round; as the length of the rope is fixed, so is the radius of the circle. At the same time, as the rope is soft, it can only provide a pulling force, which means the force is along the rope and without an angle. That is exactly like what we see in Fig. 3.2.

As long as F is perpendicular to the velocity, we will see a circle. When the magnitude of the velocity is fixed, if the force is bigger, the circle will be pulled in and become smaller. That coincides with the description of the Taiji masters who observe that when the inner power (or we may simplify it as the force) of a master gets stronger, the circle he applies becomes smaller.

So the circular movements actually signifies the spirit of Chinese martial arts — apply vertical forces and change the course of a high speed impact, "四两拨千斤."

From a more philosophical angle, the circular motion actually combines the two key principles we articulated before. As a circular motion is characterized as having one center, and all the motion happens around it, we are taking the "middle of the road" position by moving in circles.

On the other hand, circular motion is all about change: The location of the object changes, the direction of velocity changes, the direction of the acceleration changes, even the change of the acceleration changes. No wonder the Taoists love circular motions. They claim they do this because they are following the examples of the sun and the moon.

Circular motion has even more applications, which we can explain better after answering another question.

How is the Maximum Speed in a Strike Generated?

Speed comes from acceleration over time. Acceleration comes from the force we apply. Time is not within one's control in a real fight. It seems there is only one way to go: maximize the force one can apply. Following this logic, weightlifters should dominate all sports, not just fighting. But things are just not that simple.

There are actually two kind of forces in a real fight: active force and passive force.

The active force comes directly from your muscles. It is the force applied directly by the attacker at the exact time and on the exact spot controlled by the attacker. Do not be tricked by the name of the force. Active force is actually not so active. It is that kind of force you use when you lift weights in a gym following the instructions of a coach — "Do not use momentum, take it slowly up, slowly down …"

Passive force is all about momentum. It is the kind of force you feel when you are hit by a football. The football has no muscle. It is not its intention to hit you. You are hit because you are in its path trying to stop it.

In actual punching or kicking, both forces are involved. Active force is a little complicated so we will leave it for Axiom II. Passive force has three components: speed, mass, and time. It is clearly expressed by the frequently misunderstood formula below:

$$F = \Delta M / \Delta T$$

F is the passive force. M is the momentum. T is time. Δ is the standard mathematical symbol for representing change in any quantity, be it time or velocity.

As $M = mV$, so $\Delta M = \Delta(m V)$. Assume mass is a constant for a fixed object, so $\Delta M = \Delta(m V) = m \Delta V$, and we have a formula to show all the three components contributing to passive force:

$$F = m \Delta V / \Delta T$$

Contrary to conventional thinking, ΔT is not easy to control. It is mostly decided by the hardness of the materials bumping into each other. For example, the ΔT for two soft balls will be significantly bigger than two iron balls.

So the only real effective way to increase F is to increase ΔV.

To maximize ΔV, you need to have a great initial V, which is the initial velocity of the attack. If it is a punch, then it is the velocity of the fist before it hits the target.

For any single muscle system, the speed it can generate is limited. Luckily we have such a delicate but swift body to leverage.

To maximize the speed, the trick is to align the motion of all body parts and add all the velocities together. Like force, velocity is also a vector which can be added following the principle of superposition, which Galileo used to pave the path for Newton.

As shown in Fig. 3.3, there are originally three vectors, A, B, and C, shown as arrows. They add together in a tip-to-tail string and are equal to one vector A + B + C. As we can find here, the final vector A+B+C, which is the arrow from the tail of A to the tip of C, can be much longer if vector C is better aligned with vector A and B. That is exactly what we need to do in aligning the velocity of different body parts when we deliver a punch.

Now let us come back to the topic of circular motion. When we feel dazzled by the circular steps, twists, and turns of Bagua Palm, we are not even aware of the fact that basically all our movements are a combination (or superposition) of many circular or arched motions.

The fact that all our bones are rigid and bounded by joints determines that all the bones can only move around the joints. This means all our movements are arched in nature.

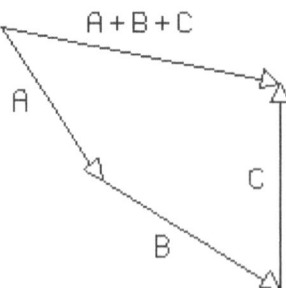

Fig. 3.3. Superposition of the velocities.

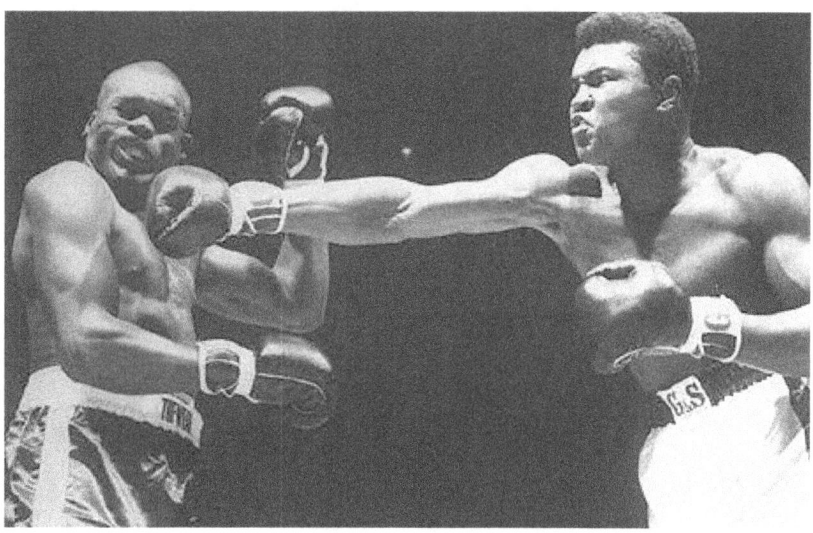

Fig. 3.4. Ali's punch.

To hit in a straight line, in this case, actually needs very sophisticated coordination among all the body parts. With the superposition principle, we will be able to add the velocities of the forward stepping, forward leaning of the whole body, the upper body turning and arm throwing into one velocity and hit the target at maximum speed.

What actually differentiates Muhammad Ali from other boxers is his quick jabs and superfast footwork, because these are the biggest elements of the final speed (Figs. 3.4 and 3.5).

The effect of superposition of the velocity can be expressed in the formula as:

$$V = V1 + V2 + V3 + V4 + \ldots + Vn$$

This can be expressed as $V = \Sigma Vn$.

It is worth noting that the major advantage of being a human in standing position is to maximize the Σ effect.

The standing position enables a vertical spin around the spine. That gives a huge leverage to combine the speed from the legs and arms to deliver speed, especially with a long stick. When you swing a very long stick, a very high speed will be generated on the tip of the stick. No wild animal can handle that kind of speed. So the correct way to handle an

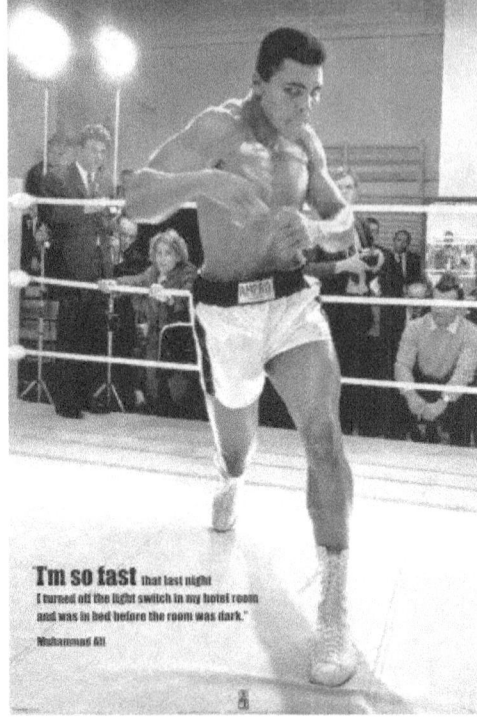

Fig. 3.5. Ali's footwork.

opponent with a bludgeon is to move in quickly before it drops, so that you will not be hit by the tip, which is most damaging.

This new type of movement not only helps to deliver higher speed but also arms us with one more dimension to change the way we move, thus making us more unpredictable in fighting.

Even the fiercest wild animals cannot perform such vertical spins as they are rooted to the ground with a horizontal spine. Can a tiger swirl? Not impossible, but very difficult indeed. That is why the Bagua Palm introduced in this book, the Weaving Stance Bagua Palm, stands out. It enables us to move like a swirling dragon flying freely in the sky, totally unpredictable and full of power.

Axiom 2: $J = \Delta F/\Delta T$ (Jing is the Real Killer)

If we vote for the most confusing concept in Chinese martial arts terminology, *Jing*（劲）will win by an unimaginable margin. It appears frequently in the martial art classics and countless articles and books, where the meaning of *Jing* is "force," yet not exactly force. In fact, it is widely used by Chinese martial artists, especially those from the inner school, to differentiate a certain force from normal force. However, this differentiation is not very successful. Most people still cannot tell the difference even after many years of martial arts training.

If you try to look for the explanation in any dictionary, you will be very disappointed. The word 劲 has two pronunciations for two meanings: *Jing* (strong) and *Jin* (force). We can even search it from the very first dictionary in China created in 100 BC — *Shuo Wen Jie Tzi* (说文解字), which was written in small seal script (an ancient Chinese script often used 2000 years ago). We will find the meaning of the word is "strong," which is the meaning of *Jing*. So, *Jing* shall be the right word. It means strong, an adjective.

Even from a Chinese martial art point of view, "force" is the word they would like to avoid to explain 劲, so we will pick *Jing* and see how we can connect it with any concept quantitatively.

Since we are developing our second axiom, we might as well follow Newton's Axiom II and see what we can find out here.

From Newton, we learn that change matters, especially change over time.

The change of location (or coordinates in mathematical terms), is the distance traveled.

The distance traveled over time is velocity.

Take location as L, time as T, and speed as V.

Change is Δ, so the location change over distance traveled is $\Delta L = L2 - L2$ (Fig. 3.6); the object is located in L1 in time T1, and it moves to L2 in time T2, so the time used for the move is $\Delta T = T2 - T1$. Now we have a simple formula:

$$V = \Delta L / \Delta T$$

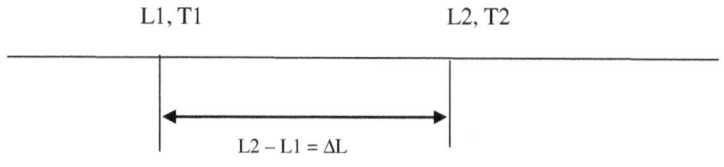

Fig. 3.6. $\Delta L = L2 - L1$

It is very easy to understand that velocity is bigger when more distance is covered in a shorter time.

Going further, we can look into the change of velocity over time.

The change of velocity over time is called acceleration, which we will take as A.

$$A = \Delta V/\Delta T$$

A is a very meaningful quantity: If the velocity changes more dramatically in a shorter time, the acceleration is very big.

Now we have already touched on Newton's Axiom II. It basically says that force is not just the reason of acceleration, it is actually proportional to it.

Thus, Newton's Axiom II states that:

$$F = mA = m\Delta V/\Delta T$$

F is the force applied to a mass, m is the quantity of the mass, and A is the acceleration caused by the force. So the force can be defined as something needed to cause change of velocity in a limited time. The greater the change of velocity, the greater the force needed; or the shorter the time allowed to make a certain change in velocity, the bigger the force needed.

Brilliant.

Let us move down further.

What is ΔA then? The change of acceleration.

How about $\Delta A/\Delta T$? What does this stand for? It looks very straightforward: the speed of acceleration change. But what does that actually mean?

There is not even an official name for that. It is called jolt, ripple, surge, lurch or mostly ... jerk. There is also not even an agreed symbol for "jerk," not because it would sound absurd, but because there are not so many direct applications for this concept.

How about adding the mass factor onto it? We all know that when mass is attached to acceleration, $mA = F$, we will get force — a much more friendly concept.

Suppose mass is a constant for the object under study, just to make it simple. Then,

$$m\Delta A/\Delta T = \Delta(mA)/\Delta T = \Delta F/\Delta T$$

Things suddenly start to become interesting from the eyes of a martial artist.

Now we have got a new concept: $\Delta F/\Delta T$, which stands for the magnitude of force changed over a limited time period. The bigger the value, the better for a fighter, as it indicates that he is more capable of changing the force (either magnitude or direction or both) he applies dramatically over a very short period of time.

This capability is a very important, if not the most important, factor in real fights.

Unlike in normal research on kinetics, where mostly only one object is studied, in a real fight, there are at least two parties involved.

Let us suppose Tom is fighting with Jerry. Both are trained fighters with the same weight, and thus, usually, similar strength. When they push or pull against each other with maximum force, we often see the fight goes nowhere. The reason is when two forces with similar magnitude go against each other, the absolute magnitude of each force is no longer important. What is important in this case is the difference between the forces, in other words, the ΔF.

This is easy to understand for a fighter. Let us suppose Jerry pushes with full strength, and he expects Tom to do the same. Tom does do the same, but only to mislead Jerry. Suddenly, Tom changes course. Instead of pushing hard, Tom pulls rapidly with a huge force. If Jerry is not able to adjust in a very short period of time, he will be thrown by Tom. As the direction of his force is the same as Tom, he has nothing to go against Tom's sudden pulling.

The scene above is often seen in wrestling. In martial arts, if Jerry can react fast, things may not go so dramatically; he may just lose his balance for a short while. Do not underestimate this short window. Because this window is created by Tom, he has a large chance to leverage it, as he actually expects it. If Tom attacks during this short window, Jerry will have a serious problem before he regains his balance.

So we can clearly see here that what is important is not the magnitude of force itself, but the newly created concept $\Delta F/\Delta T$.

This is actually where I would like the concept *Jing* (劲) to come in again. In Chinese martial art, *Jing* is usually vaguely understood as a force with intelligence. Applying *Jing* or force with intelligence means to break or defeat your opponents in the most practical and energy saving, and thus environmental friendly way.

In real fighting, especially when you are facing a trained opponent, it is very inefficient to win with pure strength, as the difference between the two of you in that regard is marginal. You will need to create a window for attack, and the window to hit is usually very narrow. A bigger ΔF and very small ΔT together make the best strategy to win. In plain words, to best explore the window, you need to change your force dramatically in the least time, that is, to apply *Jing* rather than any force without intelligence.

In traditional Chinese martial arts, *Jing* means a lot; it is not only about the speed to change force but also the speed to change body position, angle, and timing of attack.

In general, *Jing* is all about change — a typical Taoism mentality. It is the opposite of predictability. *Jing* stands for the capability to come in suddenly, to reach maximum momentum at lightning speed, and disappear like a power trip. It enables us to change directions like a snake, and to change where the attack comes from like a ghost.

Jing does not appear only in an attack. It is also used to block an attack or to create windows for attacking.

Such an all-in-one concept does have its weakness, though. As so many concepts are grouped into one, it becomes vague and difficult for analysis and causes misunderstandings, especially for the beginners.

Now we have a narrower but more accurate way to define *Jing*, which is the name of our new concept: ΔF/ΔT.

To make it official, we would like to give this new concept a symbol, *J*. Thus, $J = \Delta F/\Delta T$.

We have just wiped off the dust from a physics concept and given it a new life in not just the field of martial arts, but also in a broader field of life science. And we have even given it a name — *Jing*, together with a symbol *J*. What an achievement!

The concept of *Jing* goes beyond martial arts, in that it is connected with the way our muscles work and it enables us to understand how we can achieve better overall health.

A biological fact is that all muscles are made to shrink. That is the only way it works. Contrary to many people's beliefs, the muscle cells can apply force only in one direction: it either shrinks or relaxes. There is no other way. Because of this property, if any body part needs to be able to move in more than two directions, at least two groups of muscles need to be involved. Each time, a move to the right would need the right side of the muscle groups to shrink and pull, and at the same time, the left-side muscle groups need to relax so as not to pull too much to the left.

This is especially the case when someone is trying to find balance. The muscle groups of all sides keep on receiving instructions from the brain to shrink or relax according to the feedback from our sensory system (eyes, etc.).

When an unexpected situation happens, such as when we encounter a slippery slope, there is often very limited time for our muscles to react and adjust. In that case, those with great *Jing* will have a better chance to avoid a terrible fall. As we all know, falling-induced immobility is a common source of rapid health deterioration for the elderly. It will help this group of people greatly if we can train them to achieve better mastery of *Jing*.

Jing actually exists in all movements. Even a seemingly motionless gesture, such as holding a cup, still involves *Jing*. The muscles are made to shrink, but they are not made to hold the shrinkage for long. Even when we hold ourselves in a stationary position, our muscles are never staying "still." They just take turns to shrink and keep the position relatively stable. That is why we exhibit a little shivering when we hold a cup "still." Here, *Jing* helps us to switch between the shrink and relax status of our muscle groups.

With the understanding of *Jing*, we can try to answer some key questions, especially those related to what injures (or "damages") the human body, as a fight is all about causing and avoiding injuries to different parties.

To do that, we need to understand what the word "damage" actually means.

Geologically, to "damage" means to separate materials that used to be in one piece. This would mean to create a fracture inside materials, be it bones, muscles, or other tissues in human beings. Some fractures are obvious, such as a broken arm or leg, or a cut in the skin or muscle; some are not visible, such as a damaged organ after a heavy blow.

Many people believe that causing damage is simple — you just have to be fast enough and hit hard, that is, it all depends on velocity (V) and force (F). If that were the case, then people with a weaker body will have no chance. This is not even close to being true. It is the *Jing* that matters.

Just look at a fight between large animals, such between a lion and a buffalo. A lion can be much smaller than a buffalo and have less strength.

The lion is not even necessarily faster, but it is more capable of causing damage, not because it is faster, but because it can make sudden changes of force and has better *Jing*.

Do we have a chance facing a lion? Of course we do. A lion to us is just like a buffalo to a lion. In the end, *Jing* comes from training and intelligence. We are far better with decent training, not because we have guns, but because we are more intelligent, which enables us to have better *Jing* with proper training. Before we had guns, we had already started to dominate the earth and even driven large numbers of fierce carnivorous species into extinction.

Let us go a little deeper into the understanding of "damage." Most martial art theories touch only on the kinematics portion of physics, with some force analysis applied. However, real damage happens in materials with unique mechanical structures, such as bones, ligaments, etc. So *fracture mechanics* which includes material science and structural analysis should be an indispensable part of the study.

From the point of view of fracture mechanics, the fracturing process is an atomic-level phenomenon. A fracture happens when two layers of atoms close to each other fail to hold the bond between them. It does not really matter how big the object is or even how tough the object generally is. As long as it is solid material, the fracture is a pure local event, which happens in a range of a few rows of atoms with nearby areas involved.

Fig. 3.7 shows a giant ship broken into two pieces. The actual tear happens between the two layers of atoms of the fractured surface. The other atoms, no matter how large the number is, do not have a part in it.

Fig. 3.8 shows a schematic zoomed-in picture showing the fracture between two layers of atoms under crack-opening tension.

That is why the most "environmental friendly" way (which actually means to consume the least energy) to cause damage is to cut with a really sharp knife. A well-sharpened knife has an edge width of a few iron atoms, which is much smaller than the distance between the molecules of the skin or muscle. It can effortlessly cut through inches of skin and muscle and tissue. That is why we seldom see a surgeon sweat like a boxer does.

Anyone with some knowledge about fracture mechanics will know that fractures are not only about force — material matters, structure matters, and even time matters. A glass without a micro defect on its surface can

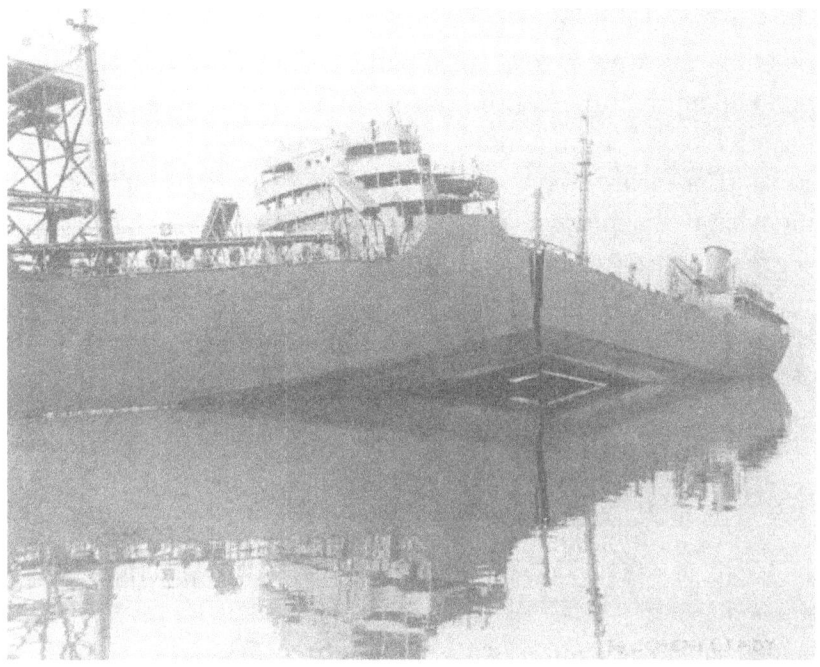

Fig. 3.7. Not exactly the *Titanic*, but still a giant ship, broken into two pieces.

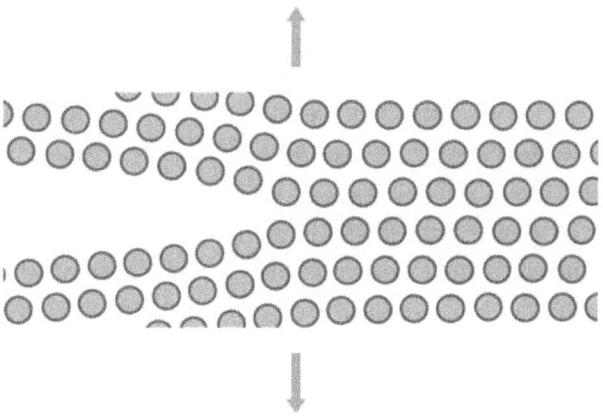

Fig. 3.8. All fractures happen in between layers of atoms.

be very strong, but it breaks easily with one-tenth the force applied when there is a scratch on its surface. A thin iron of 1mm is unbreakable with the normal force of an adult, but breaks easily in the hand of a child when he keeps on bending it back and forth (due to fatigue).

A less academic and more obvious example to illustrate the difference includes the ways we use to break a bamboo and a brick. To break a bamboo, you will apply force continuously until it bends enough to break. To break a brick, you hit it against a solid ground with a sudden force. Both bamboo and brick are easy to break if you use the right method. You can imagine what will happen if you try to break a bamboo by hitting it against a solid ground, or try to break a brick by bending it slowly.

Sun Tzu's *The Art of War* has a famous teaching which is dear to the heart of the Chinese: the first task in a war is to make yourself undefeatable. Naturally, in a real fight, the first thing is to avoid sustaining any damage before causing some. Then the question becomes:

What Helps us to Avoid Damage?

To avoid damage is the opposite of, and also the same thing as, causing damage.

We see this fact in fighters like Manny Pacquiao. He is known for his punching power and knockout record. However, few people know that he seldom suffered from any knockout in his boxing career of over 10 years.

Let us look at our body closer before the analysis. As you all know now, material science is part of the game. Although the bones are the hardest materials in our body, we are not standing strong because of the bones. A system of muscles and joints does most of the work in holding us in one piece. Without it, our bones are just a heap of loosely placed odd branches on the ground.

On the other hand, the joints and some soft parts of our body are the weak points, and thus are the targets of attacks. Knowledge about these weak points helps us to avoid suffering lethal damage. The Chinese martial art forms are partially designed for this purpose. Most of the forms ask you to place your arms around your weakest points: ear side, neck, rib area, etc. If you train yourself well, your arm will appear in those areas automatically when attacked. All this is done without thinking as we do not have the time to think under a real attack.

At the same time, the forms are very scientifically angled to shield us from attacking forces.

Remember: position, angle, and timing. We have settled the first two. Now we come to the timing part, which is trickier to understand and most difficult to master in real fighting.

Timing covers everything, even position and angle. You may start off with the right position and angle initially, but your opponent can adjust his attacking area and angle, making your position and angle ridiculous. This is the game of space adjustment. Most people will be able to learn this after some real sparring.

The timing I am trying to elaborate on here is called "inner timing." I believe that is a secret yet untold. Many people, including quite a number of martial artists, used to believe that the capability of taking a blow comes from the "toughness" of the muscles or even the skin. This is absolutely a myth.

No matter how hard you hit, rub, or move your *Qi*, flesh is flesh, and the basic physical property of the material does not change much. Do not try to convince me by showing that some "hard qigong" master can handle the chop of a broadsword. I would be much more impressed if anyone can try himself against the slide of a tiny scalpel. Skin is skin; it does not change much. Hardened skin is merely dead skin, not steel.

Then what is the real trick? The real trick is "inner timing." Let me elaborate a bit more on this new concept.

Think of our muscle cells as small liquid bags. In a relaxed state, those bags are soft and not strong enough to handle a big impact. However, when the bags shrink, the skin of these tiny bags will be much thicker and thus tougher. With the liquid inside them distributing the pressure evenly across the whole surface, the tiny bags are much stronger than we would think. If all the muscles cells shrink together, they can block and absorb very big impacts.

But no muscle is made to shrink for a long time without relaxing. That is why in real fighting, even if you have no intention to attack, it is not practical to shrink all the muscles in your body all the time and say, "I am ready to take it." You simply cannot hold this state forever. The shrink, by the nature of the muscle system, has to be short.

With that property of your muscle system in mind, the real trick has shown itself to us. The trick is not to shrink the muscles, but to shrink at the right time, and shrink together. This timing is not controlled by our thinking process, as there is obviously no time for thinking then. It is more like a built-in software in our muscle system, which signals the timing whenever it is necessary. We would like to call this inner timing.

The issue is that we are not really born with the sense of inner timing. It is acquired through training. This is where the *nei* (內 inner) *gong* (功 power) sets in.

In a Chinese martial art system, *wai* (外 outer) refers to the muscle system and *nei* (内 inner) refers to our neural system, in most cases. The *nei gong* training is the core of the inner school of martial arts. In many ways, it is similar to Yoga or any type of meditation training.

The Chinese *nei gong* training is a "tighter" process. It still involves the muscle system most of the time to build a robust link between the mind and body. In that sense, it is closer to the so-called "mindfulness" style of Yoga, as your mind never leaves your body.

However, the key of Chinese *nei gong* is to be tight and yet not too tight. This is another example of the *zhong* (中 middle of the road) way. To be tight is not to lose the connection between your mind and body. To be not too tight is not to be overly focused with your mind when practicing.

Different people may have different illusions, especially when they have worked themselves into a very deep meditation state. The right way is not to be too distracted by those illusions. Do not panic or try hard to diminish the illusions as well. You should at times have an almost "playful" attitude toward the odds in the process of tough inner strength training, which leads you to maximum power.

After we understand the mechanism of avoiding damage, we will find the next question easier:

What Makes a Chinese Martial Art Blow so Damaging?

In most cases, damage is indicated by a severe fracture, be it a bone, a patch of muscle, a tissue organ, or just the skin. A fracture that causes functional failure normally happens with a meaningful length.

As fracture involves force over a path, it is an energy-consuming phenomenon. As we understand from previous analysis, there are two kinds of forces in fighting, active and passive forces. So the energy causing the fracture also come from two sources. One is linked with the passive force, which comes basically from the kinetic energy of the attacking object. The other is linked with the active force, which mainly comes from a persistent force applied along the fracture path. This is the force that Muay Thai promotes as the "push through" force.

It also requires inner timing to apply a damaging passive force. As the formula $F = m\Delta V/\Delta T$ reveals, with the same $\Delta V/\Delta T$ value, the mass m is proportional to the passive force. Simply put, if you hit only with your fist, the power is limited. If you hit with the whole body behind the fist, the impact is much better.

For active force, inner timing is even more important, as active force is mostly applied to go against the defense of the opponent. If the opponent applies his inner timing to shrink all his muscles for defense, the attacker's inner timing needs to beat his opponent's inner timing. This will naturally require a much better mastery of *Jing* — the capability to change force in a very short period of time.

Again, the actual key point is that as the muscles are not built to shrink forever, those who master *Jing* better will be the true master of change. The master of change always wins.

As a side conclusion, we can solve the myth about what the so-called *Cun Jin* or one-inch punch that Bruce Lee popularized actually is. First of all, we shall ask ourselves a question: where is this "inch" applied? Before the punch or after it?

The answer is clear: it happens before the punch. Either because we have limited space to release the power or because we wish to make the attack more sudden and unpredictable, we apply the one-inch punch to attack whenever and wherever we want it to happen. After the punch has taken place, we should not withdraw too early. On the contrary, we would like to "push through" for maximum damage.

To maximize the punching power, we certainly want to have both active and passive forces involved. That does not mean we should confuse the active with the passive forces.

A one-inch punch is clearly an active force, which is mainly controlled by our inner timing for the suddenness of the attack. However, readers who know some physics but are not really good at it often get confused by the formula we introduced earlier:

$$F = m\Delta V/\Delta T$$

Based on the formula, they conclude, the time of velocity change should be as short as possible to maximize the force. So if they were fighting, they would quickly withdraw their fist right after they hit their opponent to "minimize the time." The result is that their opponent will not be impressed with their "inch punching" power at all.

Their mistake lies in the fact that this formula is for describing the mechanism of generating passive force, but "inch punching" is mainly active force. The "inch" here refers to the distance before the punch happens, not after it.

Axiom 3: The Δ and Σ Both Come from Your Liver

Now we know clearly that a powerful attack usually involves both active force and passive force.

The passive force alone can be very powerful if applied properly. However, it is not always convenient in a real fight to apply passive force, as it involves kinetic energy that takes some time to generate. However, applying force perpendicular to the velocity can change the direction of the passive impact effectively and make it an effective weapon against opponents.

The circular motion comes in here with great value. When you move in circles, there will not be a point in time where your velocity becomes zero. Thus the kinetic energy either generated by you from previous moves or gotten directly from your opponent comes in handy for you to apply whenever you need it.

The active force, on the other hand, is capable of causing serious damage with minimum energy consumed while applying the *Jing*. However, *Jing* is a very difficult skill to master. And the fact that the effectiveness of *Jing* applied is dependent on the inner timing skill makes it even tougher, as inner timing is another difficult skill to master.

Those who master *Jing* have great capability to apply significant force in no time. They are capable of breaking their opponent's defense built on the reaction triggered by their inner timing skills. Those attacked by *Jing* will experience extreme shock like a whiplash.

It might actually make great sense to refer back to the original meaning of *Jing*, which is to be strong. Martial artists who have mastered *Jing* are actually stronger than strong, because being strong does not secure victory all the time, whereas those with great *Jing* win all the time. They are more alive than alive, because in their eyes, the opponents are not just weaker or slower, but simply as dead as a piece of meat on the chopping board.

The method of obtaining maximum active force is to apply *Jing* triggered by inner timing, which is all about the positive Δ of the forces.

The method of obtaining maximum passive force is to align the velocities of different parts of the body, which is all about the Σ of the velocities.

As we all know, Δ and Σ are very different operations. The mysterious part is we can coordinate them at the same time with our Yi (意mind).

Yi is actually another tricky concept in Chinese martial arts, only next to Jing. Yi is often interpreted as mind, but it is actually between mind and mindless.

Yi is not a product of our brain or our heart, as the two were regarded as the same most of the time in the Chinese martial arts dictionary. It certainly does not come from our feet as the Xingyi puts it — 消息全凭后足蹬; the message is sent by the push-off of the foot from behind. Then it has to come from somewhere in the middle. I want to assign it to Dan Tian (丹田) — which to me is actually the center of gravity of our body. However, not many people know what that is, so why not just assign it to the liver? It is big enough to be very important and it is quite solid and God knows what is inside — mysterious!

It seems to me that it does make great sense that people name it "liver" with the belief that there is a lot of vitality stored inside it. Actually those who have mastered Yi will be able to have powerful Jing and perfect coordination, which do make people more "alive" than normal people, like a leopard in a herd of sheep.

The Yi might not be the source of Jing, but it surely is the controller of it. The trick about applying Yi is trickier than Yi itself — just like keeping a cat at home: you should not ignore it, but you should not be too keen to control it, either!

The good news is, however tricky it is, like any other martial art form, we can master it through continuous practicing, and practice makes perfect. Chinese martial art is not something you can learn by reading and thinking only. It is an art you need to learn with your body. You will learn actually nothing without involving your body.

In the process of practicing and learning Chinese martial art, you will find the boundary between your mind and body gradually dissolving. Eventually it would even be hard to identify whether Jing and Yi are from our mind or our body. One day, you would find yourself thinking with your body and moving with your mind. This is not even remotely scientific, but I am not exactly joking.

This type of expression is typical in many Chinese martial art classics. It is essentially like a painting from Picasso (Fig. 3.9). You do not expect the actual world to look remotely like what he has painted, but he is not a lunatic; he is trying to express something in a unique way.

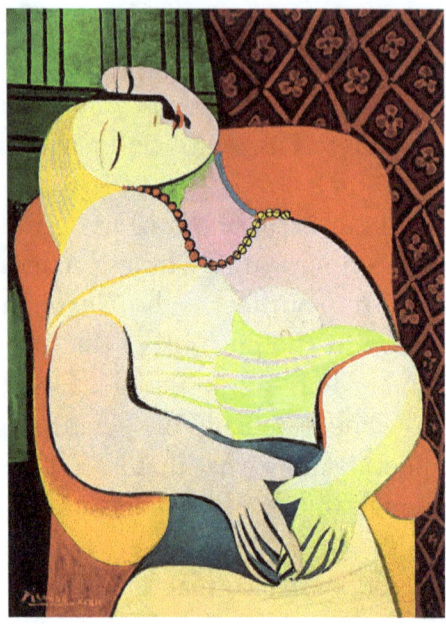

Fig. 3.9. One of Picasso's masterpieces.

(As I was writing this part of the book, something interesting happened. Just less than 10 hours after I wrote the paragraph above, I looked at my mobile phone and saw that somebody had quoted Picasso: "Art is a lie that makes us realize truth." I had never heard of this quote before I wrote that paragraph about Picasso! Talk about coincidence!)

This is the end of my Axiom III. It actually looks more like half of an axiom from the angle of scientific rigor. Besides the level of difficulty of the topic itself, it is purposely done that way. As a student of physics, I wish to show some respect to Isaac Newton by not pretending to be his equal … at least, not in this book!

Part II: Taoism in Action: The 64 Forms of Bagua Palm

When asked by his student what he was actually good at, Mencius, the second-greatest master in Confucianism, replied, "I am good at cultivating my mighty Qi."

Notice the verb he used: "cultivating," not "gathering" or "training." Probably because the Chinese martial arts have been developed in the period when farming culture was largely dominant in China, cultivating has always been a core concept in Chinese martial arts.

Cultivating is not only a different concept from training, but it is also almost a concept contradictory to training. Two seemingly contradictory items can form the simplest cycle. The cultivating and training cycle forms the major activity of Chinese martial arts.

Cultivating as part of a farming culture has certain traits that are rare in a nomadic culture. In nomadic cultures, the focus is on seizing more resources, and radical actions are necessary at times. In farming cultures, the focus is on making the best use of the existing resources. Cultivating is thus a core element of the farming culture.

In the process of cultivating, you do not just do whatever you want at your own pace. Instead, the key is to follow the rhythm of nature, to do what is necessary and wait for things to happen. Obviously, in agriculture, it is not advised to pull the plants to make them grow faster.

The same attitude applies to the exercise of Bagua Palm. As a Taoist martial art, Bagua should not be performed with too much force and power, especially in the beginning stages, or you risk never getting its essence. In addition to your body needing to stay relaxed, your mind shall stay calm as well.

Many martial art enthusiasts are in favor of physical challenges. To them, it is almost frustrating to be asked not to apply too much force in training. Actually, a large part of the reason not to apply too much force is that force is the reason for wrong stances. Without force, many bad habits are just unsustainable. Try to maintain an unnatural stance without applying force, and you will know it is impossible.

It is important to get the stances and forms right, especially at the beginning stage. However, it is even more important to relax your mind. If you do every stance and form right, but with a wrong mindset, such as a highly nervous mind, everything will go wrong. That is the tricky part of Chinese inner martial arts.

The most common mistake for beginners is to learn too much too soon from the beginning. They stress themselves out by remembering all the key points of the movements, the sequences, and the changes in a short time. In the end, they get too nervous to grasp the spirit of the style.

That is the reason why less is more while learning and practicing the inner school of Chinese martial arts. The emperors of the Qing dynasty used to have small chambers in their palaces with even the sizes of the furniture suitable for only one person. Obviously it was not because the emperors could not afford bigger rooms and bigger furniture. They were practicing the principle of less is more.

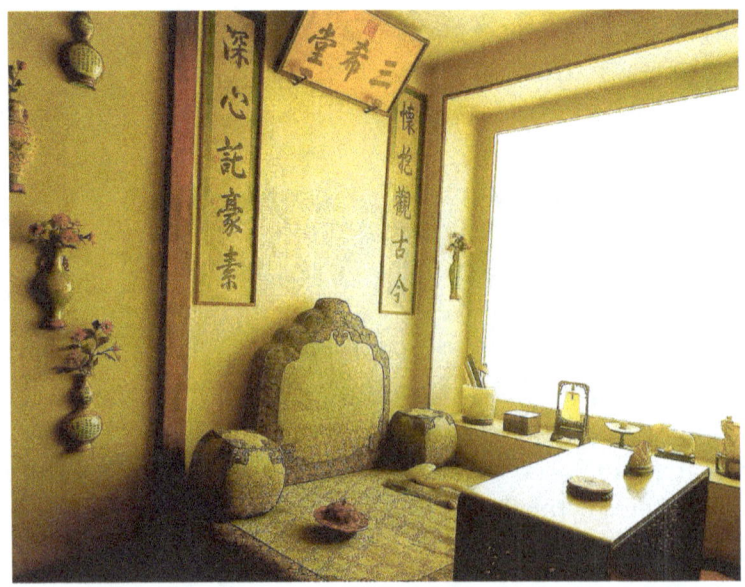

养心殿 The Palace of Mental Cultivation, the Forbidden City, Beijing, China.

This simplicity served a single purpose: to help the emperors enjoy solitude and find peace of mind, thus the name of the palace — the Palace of Mental Cultivation — *Yang* (养 cultivate) *Xin* (心 heart) *Dian* (殿 palace).

For the Chinese, health is not one word but the combination of two characteristics — *Jian*健*Kang*康 — *Jian* means a strong body, and *Kang* means a delighted heart (体壮曰健, 心怡曰康).

So always keep this in mind: Bagua is not merely an exercise of the body but also of the mind, and as in all other inner styles of martial arts, the mind and body are one. When you apply your mind, or so-called *Yi*, try not to use too much "force" as well. The more you push your mind, the further away you will be from the *Tao*.

It takes time to finish the process of joining the body and mind into one. So, do not hurry or worry, but be happy.

4
Basic Principles for Practicing Bagua Palm

As the most recently created form of Chinese martial arts, Bagua Palm (Fig. 4.1) absorbed most key principles from all other schools, including the outer schools of Chinese martial arts. To be frank, those common principles actually form the majority of all the rules a Bagua student will follow. If the whole universe is created from one *Tao*, how different can two martial art styles be essentially?

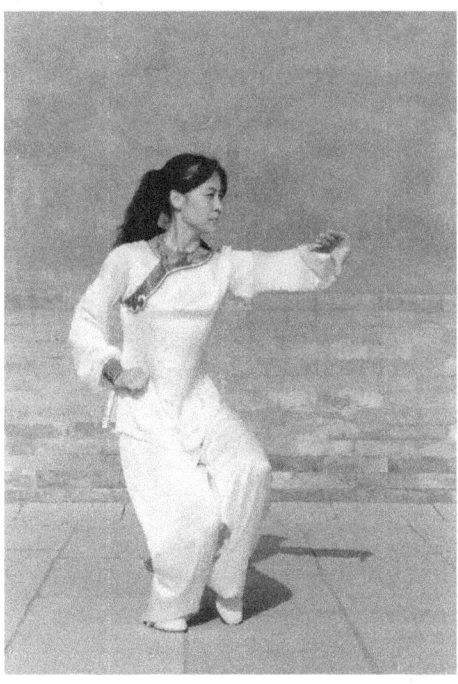

Fig. 4.1. 八卦掌 — Bagua Palm performed by Master Ge Chun Yan.

On the other hand, learners from different levels of study do need quite different instructions from the masters. Actually, the requirements for people from different levels in the same style should be different, while what is required of people at similar levels from different schools of martial arts should be more or less similar.

A martial art is an art of body practice. If they rationalize the process too much but don't practice enough, it is almost impossible for beginners to even understand what is required, let alone grasp the moves.

To avoid accidents, normal Chinese martial art systems typically introduce sparring at a fairly late stage of study. However, without real fighting experience, many of the forms and techniques simply go misunderstood in the teaching process.

The danger of setting rules for practicing lies in the fact that people tend to overdo it when they are required to follow certain rules, especially when they are beginners. When asked not to use too much force in practicing, many behave as if they are affected by myasthenia gravis; when asked to maintain an upright position, they become as stiff as puppets.

This is the most difficult part of martial art education. The teaching has to be tailor-made according to each student's situation or it will lose most of its effectiveness.

In this chapter, we will try to do the impossible: list out the do's and don'ts of practicing Bagua and hope it works.

We will also use more pictures to illustrate the points. A picture is worth more than a thousand words, especially when the topic is action science.

Some do's:

1. Stay in middle of the road and stay vigilant with a mind ready to change.

As we showed it in Chapter Two, if you do not know enough, stay in the middle. On the other hand, nothing can go seriously wrong if you are able to change and adjust.

2. Be happy.

Everything will be fine as long as you are happy. Often, when you are grumpy, things just naturally go unnaturally wrong. So, go practice with a smile on your face.

Figure 4.2 shows the famous calligraphy masterpiece, the Chives, by top calligrapher Yang Ning Shi from over 1000 years ago. It is ranked as

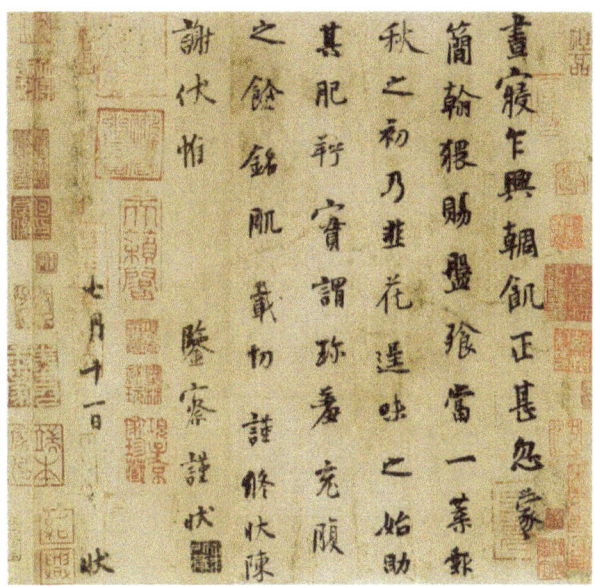

Fig. 4.2. The fifth best calligraphy artwork of all time — the Chives 韭花贴.

the fifth best calligraphy piece in history by some experts. The spirit we see from this masterpiece is what we want to achieve in practicing Bagua — joyousness, effortless control of distances, well-balanced and coordinated moves, utmost resourcefulness, and mindfulness of the big picture, much more than words can convey.

The best advice I have ever seen about practicing inner school Chinese martial arts comes from master Sun Lu Tang in his book, *The Edited Conversations on Bagua Palms*, which is not just simple and straightforward but also close to complete.

Some don'ts :

1. Do not be angry.

There is a Chinese saying which states that anger will overwhelm thinking capability, which means anger will prevent you from thinking clearly. Only when your mind is clear can you keep alert about the adjustments necessary according to the changing situations.

2. Do not apply mindless force.

Applying mindless force in martial arts brings you nothing except getting your muscles exhausted. Worse, when this becomes an ingrained habit through years of wrong practice, it totally excludes you from mastering the ultimate skill in martial arts — the ability to master a change of forces in a very limited time to gain *Jing*.

Mindless workouts make the muscles stiff and will hurt the blood circulation in the end. Be mindful when you move and stay alert with a mind for change.

3. Do not stick out your chest or belly.

The stiffness you create around your chest or belly will block the flow of *Qi* between your upper body and lower body. It also renders poor coordination between your body parts and hurts your balancing capability. You will be easily lifted up or knock down in actual fighting.

Here are nine key points to take note of:

1. *Ta* (塌)

This is about the waist, which has to sink down as if something is collapsing (Fig. 4.3). At the same time, the lower end of the spine should be lifted up slightly, not forcefully, but controlled with your mind.

This is to make sure that the *Du* (督) Meridian, which is basically the channel for *Qi* running up from the back of the body, is kept open.

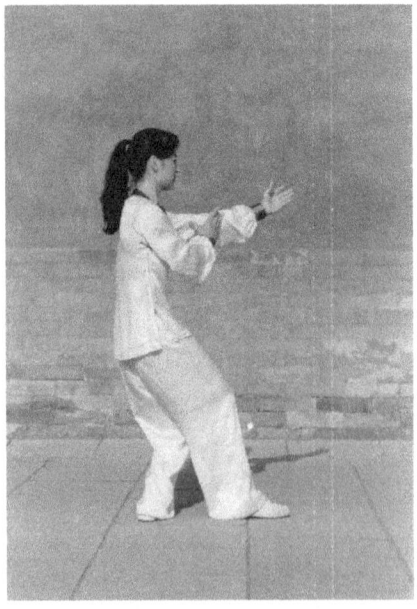

Fig. 4.3. *Ta.*

2. *Kou* (扣)

This is basically the opposite of sticking out your chest or belly. The shoulders should also slightly fold forward and form a C-shape when viewed from the top (Fig. 4.4). This is to relax the belly so as not to block the *Qi* flow in the *Ren* (任) Meridian, which is basically the channel for *Qi* running down from the front of the body.

This will make the upper body look like a shallow bowl. The same shape applies to the hands and feet. This will make the hands and feet relaxed and yet ready for releasing power.

The third part of Kou requires the teeth to bite slightly. Do bear in mind that all these *Kou* shall not be done with much actual force, but rather, with your mind. Otherwise, you might as well forget about it, as in this case, too much is worse than none.

3. *Ti* (提)

Ti is to lift up the perineum area, again, slightly without using much force. It is more or less like you are trying to hold back your urination.

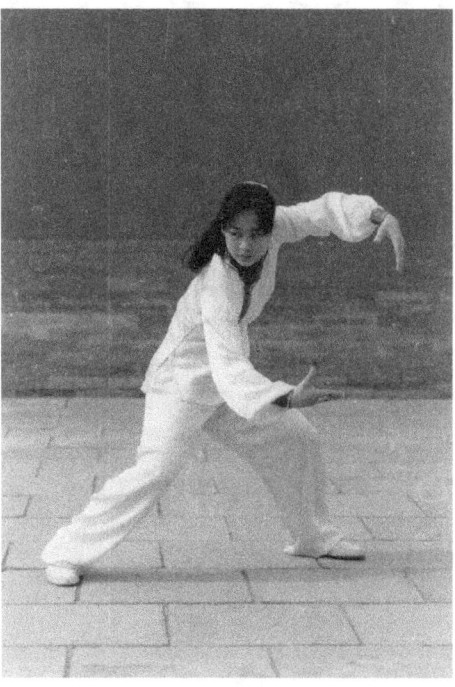

Fig. 4.4. *Kou.*

This is one of the typical inner style trainings with no change of outlook, but rather that applies the *Yi*, or mind, to enhance our inner spirit.

4. *Ding* (顶)

There are three parts to this action.
> First, keep the tongue touching the palate.
> Second, keep the neck straight up as if carrying something on the head.
> Third, maintain a pushing-forward intention with both hands (Fig. 4.5).

5. *Suo* (缩)

Suo is to have the intention to withdraw from the hipbones and the shoulders (Fig. 4.6). *Suo* is the opposite of Ding but applies on different parts of the body. It forms a tension in the arms and legs to help stretch the tendon and enable *Jing* to release faster.

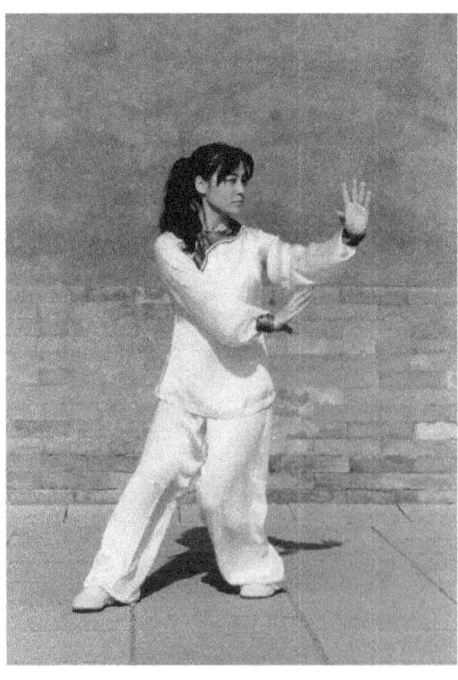

Fig. 4.5. *Ding.*

Basic Principles for Practicing Bagua Palm   71

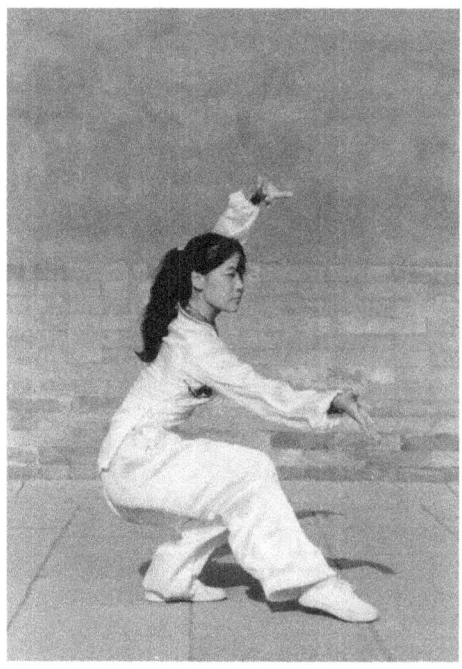

Fig. 4.6. *Suo*.

6. *Song* (松)

Song means to relax the shoulders (Fig. 4.7).

7. *Chui* (垂)

Chui is to maintain a pointing-downward intention with the tips of the elbows (Fig. 4.8).

8. *Guo* (裹)

Guo is to maintain a wrapping-upward intention with both elbows, as if holding something up (Fig. 4.9).

9. Be clear about *Qi* (起 raise) *Zuan* (钻 pierce) *Luo* (落 drop) *Fan* (翻 turn)

This part is about attacking with arms and hands. *Qi* and *Zuan* means to raise the arms and pierce forward. *Luo* and *Fan* means to drop arms for interdiction with inward turning of the forearm (Fig. 4.10).

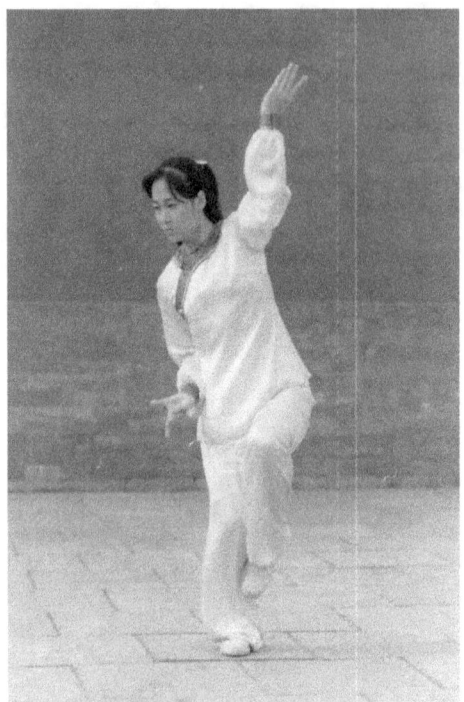

Fig. 4.7. *Song.*

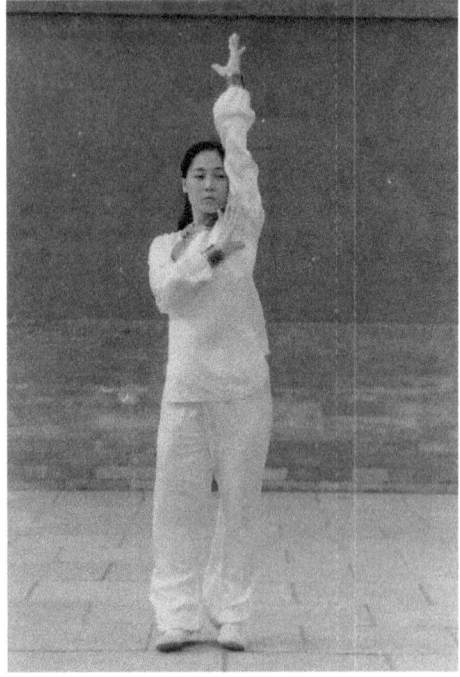

Fig. 4.8. *Chui.*

Basic Principles for Practicing Bagua Palm 73

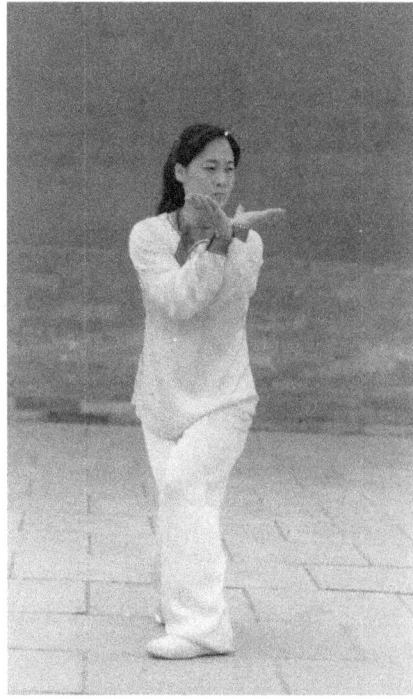

Fig. 4.9. *Guo.*

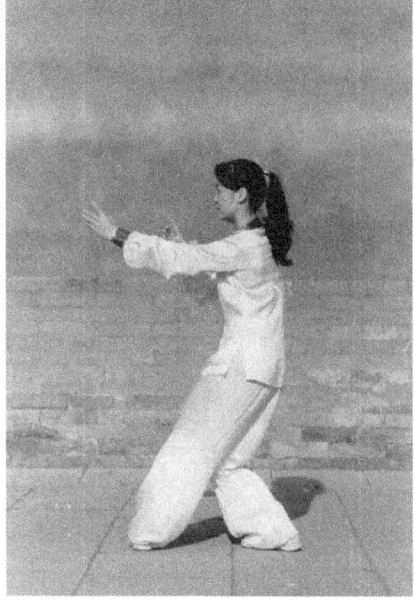

Fig. 4.10. *Qi Zuan* and *Luo Fan*.

Raising and piercing is one action; dropping and turning is another action. In actual fighting, these actions may not appear exactly in turn, and the difference in speed and rhythm may blur. However, in practicing, these two actions should be performed with clear-cut difference in a more or less fixed manner. This will help the body to remember the rhythm and achieve better coordination.

This might be a bit confusing for those without fighting experience. For the experts, however, the reason is very straightforward. A real fight is messy. There are just too many variables, with instant changes to make. Only when you build up a solid norm in practice can you eliminate the unnecessary changes and leave room for important changes needed in actual fighting.

There are three important footwork steps for Bagua that all practitioners should master: mud-wading steps (the whole of Chapter 5 is dedicated to this topic), *Kou* steps, and *Bai* steps.

Mud-wading steps are the fundamentals of the whole Bagua system. This topic is too important to be mixed with other forms. So it merits an entire chapter to itself. People who have no interest in the self-defense applications of Bagua can actually skip most of the contents of this book and go straight to Chapter 5 for great wellness enhancement values.

Both *Bai* and *Kou* steps have the function of locking the legs of the opponents as well as changing directions of the body. In a way, without *Bai* and *Kou*, the path of the Bagua movements will become a straight line rather than a serious of curves or circles.

As Figs. 4.11 and 4.12 show, *Bai* and *Kou* are opposite to each other in terms of the direction the foot points.

Bai is often used to move to the outer side of the opponent to avoid being attacked. When walking in a circle, the foot close to the center of the circle will move straight, while the other foot will move in a *Kou* way.

With the direction change of the steps following *Bai* or *Kou*, the body also turns or twists around the spine. This is a movement unique to Man, which adds a new dimension of change in terms of position, speed, and force. At the same time, it can maximize the possible speed of attack from a totally unforeseeable angle. All these give Man extra advantage over even the fiercest carnivores.

From the wellness point of view, there is a *Dai* channel which surrounds us in the waist area like a belt. The *Dai* channel will be trained by

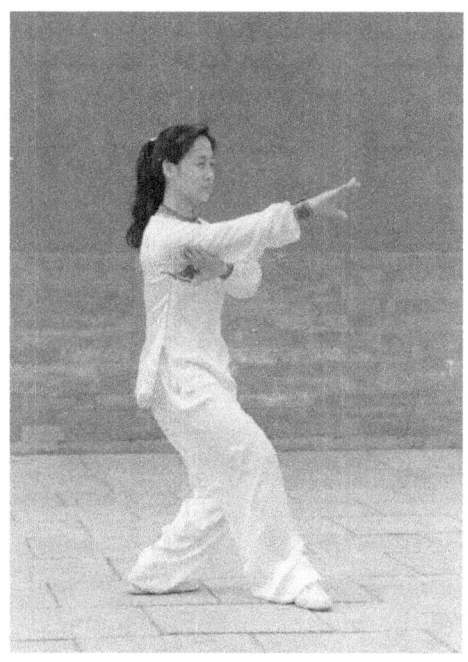

Fig. 4.11. *Bai.*

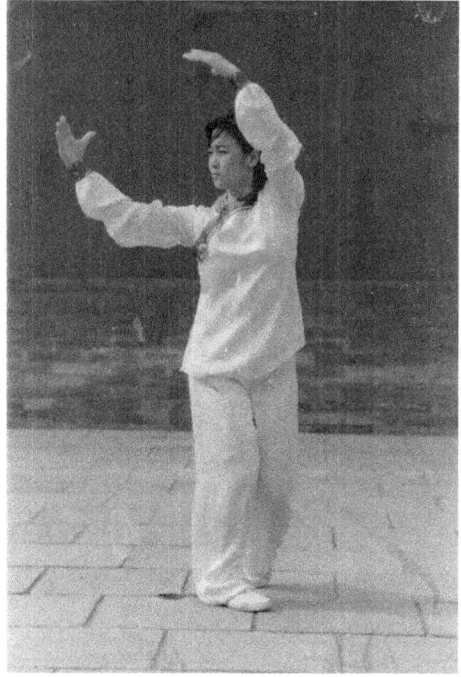

Fig. 4.12. *Kou.*

the frequent turning around of the vertical spine while practicing Bagua Palm's *Bai* and *Kou* steps.

As master Cheng Ting Hua was a wrestler before learning Bagua, the *Kou* step was used by him to lock the front leg of the opponent while closing in, thus the name inward-latching step.

For every step in Bagua, the toes need to grasp the ground with the center of the foot drawn up in mind, while focusing on the center of the bottom of the foot (*yong quan*) to move the *Qi* there.

For the shape of the palms, the Cheng School applies a typical dragon claw (龙爪掌), as we can see from Fig 4.13. The thumbs and index fingers open wide, and the rest of the fingers are close to each other. As stressed before, all the fingers bend and form a cup shape, as if holding a basketball.

Bagua treats the whole body as a connected system with the reference of the ancient Chinese medical theories. The ancient Chinese treated the body as a network of the Meridians and channels through which the *Qi* runs all over the body.

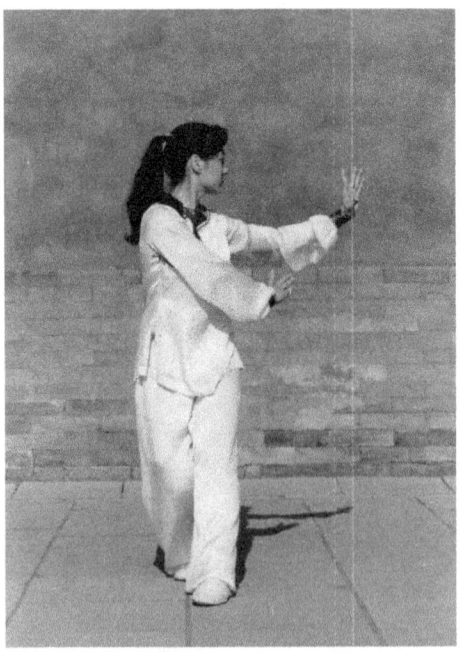

Fig. 4.13. The dragon claw.

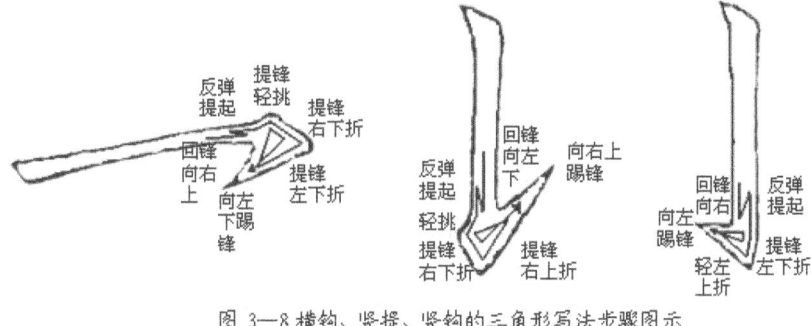

Fig. 4.14. The reverse movements of the strokes.

In the first chapter of the ancient Chinese medical book *Huangdi Neijing (The Yellow Emperor's Outer Canon)*, it was mentioned that the ancient Chinese used to "move with the heaven and earth, master *Yin* and *Yang* (change), breathe the spirit and *Qi*, stand alone with the mind guiding the body, and make the muscles of whole body as one (提挈天地, 把握阴阳, 呼吸精气, 独立守神, 肌肉若一。)."

This is a great description of the movements of Bagua Palm, where one seeks movements in stillness and pushes arms forward with a mind to withdrawing them, so as to preserve a sense of contradiction in movements which keeps the body alert for any changes necessary. At the same time, the stress created from the contradictions will work to keep the whole body as a well-unified body of full mindfulness.

In a way, the movement of inner school martial arts is similar to Chinese calligraphy, in that all the strokes need to firstly move to the opposite direction before they start to move in a planned direction (Fig. 4.14). No wonder when asked by his grandchild why he kept on practicing calligraphy rather than martial arts, Sun Lu Tang replied, "I am actually practicing the sword!"

5
The Mud-Wading Steps

There is a well-known saying in Chinese martial arts: "Walking is the basis of all forms and its effectiveness beats hundreds of forms."

If we apply the methodology of superposition principles, a typical martial art movement can be separated into at least four levels of movements with different magnitude and nature (Fig. 5.1).

For example, the movement shown in Fig. 5.2 involves two steps to the left in an arc.

The first-order approximation is a translational motion which only changes the position of an object. This is actually mostly walking (Fig. 5.3).

The second-order approximation is the rotation of the main body, which only changes the direction of an object (Fig. 5.4).

The third-order approximation is the stretch of legs and arms (Fig. 5.5).

The normally neglected "smaller" movements of wrists and fingers, which is very important for Cheng Style Bagua with its many catching and wrestling techniques, can be classified as the fourth-order approximation.

Needless to say, as the first-order movement, walking involves the most energy and creates the biggest change in distance. It is thus the most significant and most effective movement in martial arts.

In other words, walking is the foundation of any sports on the ground. If you want to win it, clearly good footwork is a must. If we watch a boxing match, we can see that a simple sidestep can have significant consequences and completely change the situations of the boxers. It can make any move of the opponent look ridiculous. It is much more effective than many dazzling arm waving and blocking techniques. Hence, footwork is the first thing a serious martial art student should master.

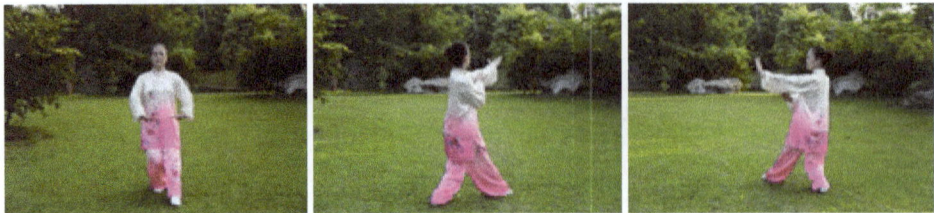

Fig. 5.1. A typical Bagua starting movement.

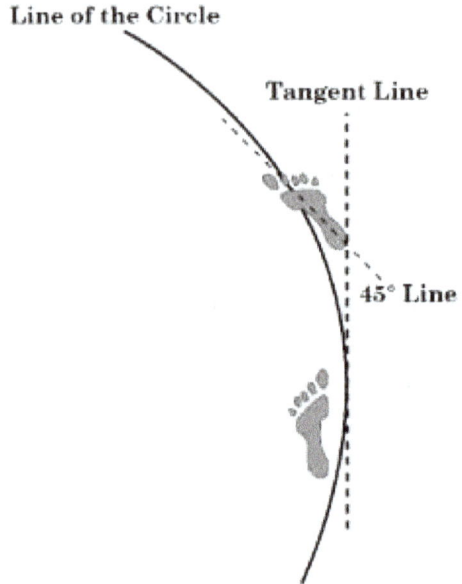

Fig. 5.2. Track on the ground.

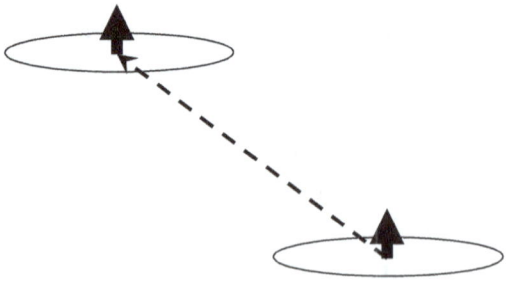

Fig. 5.3. Location change of the object.

 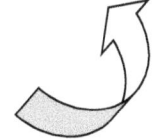 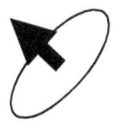

Fig. 5.4. Direction change of the object.

 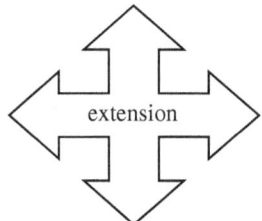 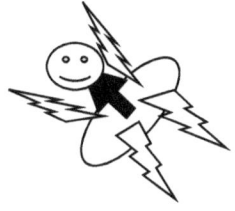

Fig. 5.5. Extension change of the object.

Bagua Palm is first of all a martial art famous for swift footwork, while the mud-wading steps are the symbolic steps of Bagua. It includes most of the rules governing the movements of body and mind in practicing Bagua. Naturally, if you get the mud-wading steps right, you have gotten the bigger part of Bagua right.

From the standpoint of enhancing power, mud-wading steps represent a basic and effective method. In terms of muscle power, wading can help you increase the strength of your waist and legs quickly and you will feel very well rooted when standing. It trains you to maintain a peaceful mind not only when you are motionless but also when you are moving. You will be able to keep yourself in one united body with a focused mind by imaginatively sinking your *Qi* into the lower belly area. Your fighting skill only matters when you can hold yourself in one piece while fighting.

So, wading should be the first Bagua move that you start practicing, and it is a skill you will keep on honing all your life.

Key Points for the Mud-Wading Steps

According to Grand Master Sun Zhi Jun, the most respected master alive of the Cheng School Bagua, the wading steps involve walking forward as if wading through shallow water and landing the foot as if on mud. So while landing, the toes need to grasp the ground as if to prevent sliding.

To walk forward as if wading through shallow water means to keep a narrow gap between the sole and the ground. The movement is like using your sole to rub and roll a cord on the ground. To land the foot as if on mud means to step firmly and carefully with the toes grasping the ground for better stability, always being alert and maintaining the capability to react quickly in case of possible sliding and other sudden situations.

It is worth noting that there is some misunderstanding about the requirement to "lift flat and land flat" while performing the wading steps. The actual meaning is to maintain the level of the center of gravity as a whole when stepping out and landing the feet. Some people read that as a requirement to keep the soles of both feet parallel to the ground at all times no matter whether you are moving out or landing. That is very unnatural and has been proven to be almost impossible.

The major type of wading exercise is called Yong (涌surge) step. The requirement is to keep the instep of the front foot naturally straight while moving forward so as not to stress the ankle. When the front leg is straight, push off the back leg to make the front foot "surge" forward for a certain distance.

The forward stepping needs to be performed continuously while keeping the sole of the forefoot parallel to the ground with a small gap. The smaller the gap the better, but never touch the ground before landing. Always go straight when moving forward for the shortest distance. Figure 5.6 shows the route you should take – route C.

The toes should grasp the ground while landing the foot and keeping the center of gravity of your body toward the back as if sitting on something.

This way of walking is not only fast but also is less stressful for the ankle, which allows you to walk for a longer time. The front foot is faster

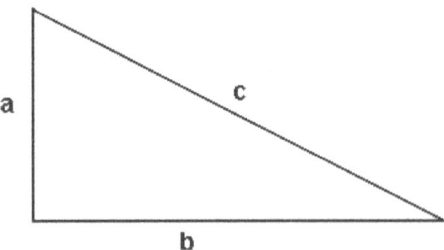

Fig. 5.6. a + b > c.

and similar to running while the leg behind is more like walking; the two feet coordinate to move forward. But never jump or leap, otherwise it will be hard to keep the *Qi* downward to maintain stability. Do not raise the foot too high or the speed will be lost.

The stance has similar requirements to that covered in Chapter 4. Keep the neck straight up as if carrying something on the head (as in the *Ding* stance). The shoulders should form a shallow C. Tighten the back and loosen the chest to form a C for the upper body, sinking down the waist and hipbones. Do not hump the back or stick out the hips. Maintain a general vertical and upright body stance, keeping the center of gravity on the back leg most of the time.

Be smooth and uniform in speed while walking. Maintain the same height of the body and avoid sudden changes in speed and up-and-down movements of the body.

Breathe naturally with the tongue touching the palate. Imagine sinking the *Qi* into the lower belly, while loosening the belly muscle and feeling the natural surging of the *Qi* inside it. Keep the two legs close to the central line while walking.

There are three different stances of different body heights to choose while walking. The upper stance is the natural height while walking, the mid stance is slightly squatted, and the lower stance is to have the hip at the same height as the knee — do not go any lower than this.

A Detailed Illustration of Mud-Wading Steps

The mud-wading steps enable a fighter to attack like a dragon and disappear like a ghost in front of the enemy. As a beginner of Bagua Palm, it is very hard to master mud-wading steps to that level no matter how much experience you have had in other martial arts. Because Bagua is such a unique martial arts with a unique philosophy and norms, it is almost a torture trying to get it right at the beginning.

Many would feel discouraged and ask themselves, *How can one master such a complicated system when even the beginning stage is so difficult?* However, the good news is, mastering the mud-wading steps is actually almost the most difficult part; once you have mastered it, the rest of the forms, no matter how complicated they look, will become much easier. So be patient and pay extra attention to practicing the mud-wading steps and you will have solid fundamentals for the whole Bagua system.

The teaching methodology of the wading steps shown here is summarized by Master Ge Chun Yan, based on the rigorous and meticulous training method of the official Beijing Martial Arts Team, where many of the most influential martial artists such as Jet Li and Donnie Yen came from. It also includes the teaching of numerous grand masters of Chinese martial arts all over China and the experience she gained from teaching practitioners, both professionals and new students in the field. This is the first time she has put this proven methodology into print.

First Step: Wading in a Straight Line Without Arm Movements

It is easier to start from a straight line rather than a circle to learn the wading steps.

First, place the hands at the waist, standing with feet next to each other. Then bend the legs to lower the center of gravity and relax. This will be the level of your center of gravity in the whole process (Fig. 5.7).

Move the right foot forward with the sole parallel to the ground, keeping the center of gravity with the left leg. Keep pushing off with the left

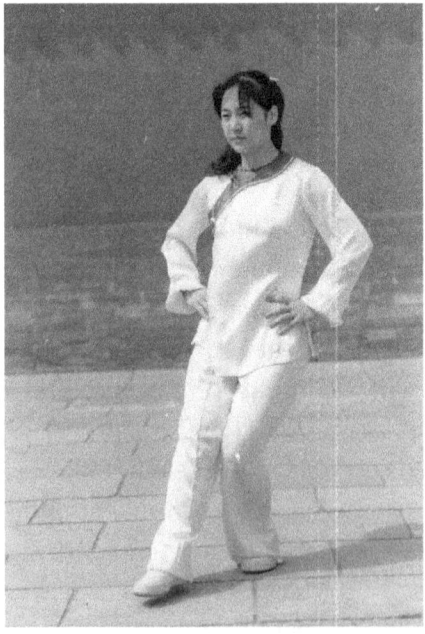

Fig. 5.7. Master Ge Chun Yan demonstrating mud-wading steps.

leg to drive the right foot forward. Once the right foot has landed, start to shift the body weight to the right leg and then lift the left foot and prepare to step forward. Keep the sole of the left foot parallel to the ground while lifting.

Next, step forward with the left foot, passing the right foot closely and keeping the sole parallel and close to the ground. The stepping forward of the front foot and pushing off of the back leg should take place at the same time to maintain a uniform rhythm while keeping the body upright.

Keep your mind relaxed and body upright, be fluid and smooth in your movements, and maintain a uniform rhythm. These requirements will help the *Qi* to sink into the lower belly — the *Dan Tian* — which is very important in inner martial arts.

Through the straight line wading practice, we are able to focus on the stability of the center of gravity, keeping the legs bent all the time at the same level and soles parallel to the ground while moving ahead. It is also easier to achieve stability while moving even when the two legs and feet are so close to each other as to almost rub each other while crossing. After all the requirements are achieved, we can move on to the next level, the circular wading.

Second Step: Circular Wading

Circular movements are more typical in Bagua. As the left and right sides are no longer symmetric in circular wading, balance and coordination are a major focus.

1. Preparatory posture

Stand up naturally with the feet close to each other, head and neck upright, chest and abdomen relaxed with the shoulders hanging down loosely, arms hanging beside the thighs, palms relaxed and facing inward naturally. Breath naturally, keeping the eyes level, and stay focused (Fig. 5.8).

2. Spread arms upward

Raise both arms from the side of the body until level with the shoulders, palms facing upwards (Fig. 5.9).

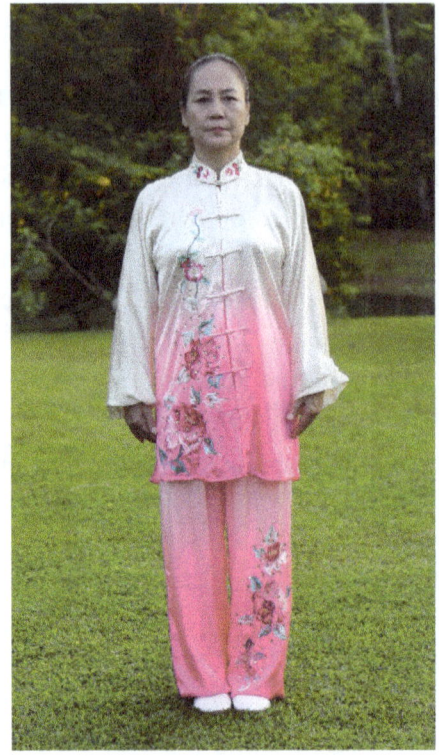

Fig. 5.8. Preparatory posture.

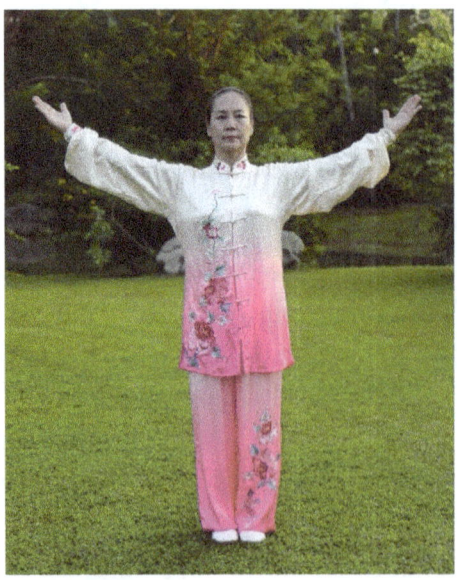

Fig. 5.9. Spread arms upward.

3. Fold arms

Turn the palms facing down, folding the arms to the same width as the shoulder and holding the hands in front of the chest close to each other (Fig. 5.10).

4. Push palms downward

While squatting down slowly, push both palms downward until they reach the front of the lower abdomen. While you do this, feel the *Qi* sinking into the lower abdomen. Lean slightly backward with the neck upright. Keep the arms curved and upper body straight and grip the ground solidly with the toes while leaving the center part of the soles slightly away from the ground to provide a sort of sucking intension (Fig. 5.11).

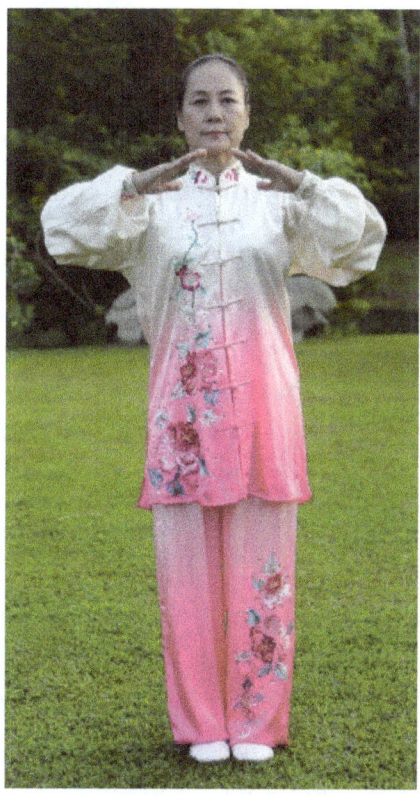

Fig. 5.10. Fold arms.

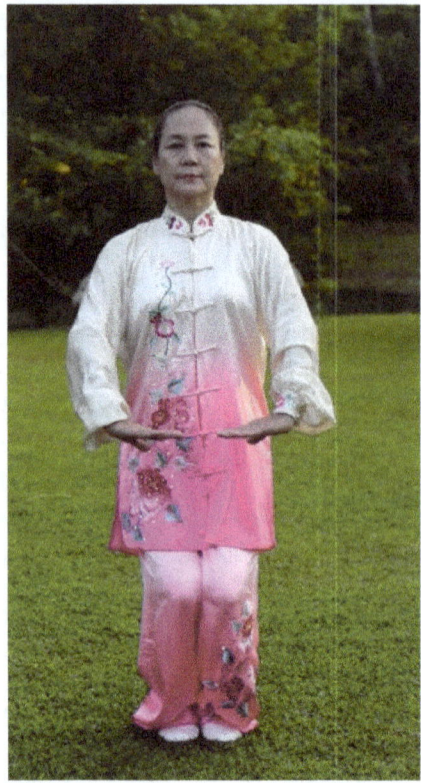

Fig. 5.11. Push palms downward.

5. Step forward

Lift the left leg and wade forward, with the sole parallel to the ground, letting the body's center of gravity sit on the right leg. The left foot should move forward further before it lands (Fig. 5.12). While placing down the left foot, push the ground with your right leg and start to move forward with your right foot. The center of gravity will then be shifted to the left leg. Then move the right foot forward further. When the right foot is lifted, move forward, holding the toes back slightly to maintain the horizontal position of the sole to the ground.

Move the right leg forward along the right side of the left foot, letting the tip of the right foot swing slightly to the left, and wade forward slightly toward the left side. The sole should be maintained parallel to the ground while moving forward. When the front leg lands, the back leg forcefully

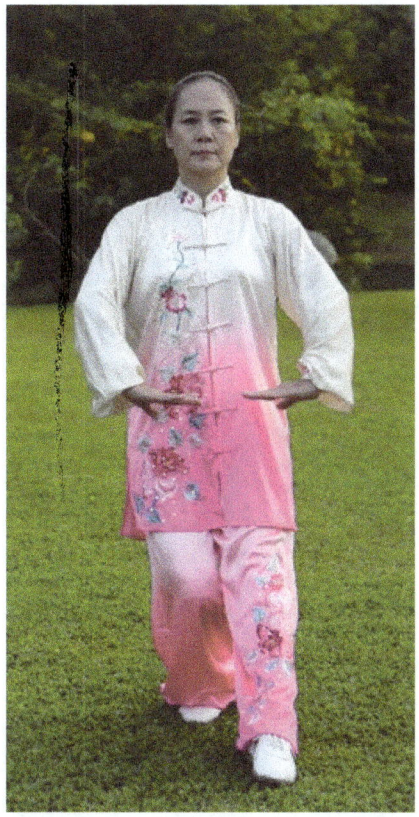

Fig. 5.12. Take the first step forward.

pushes the ground backward at the same time. Maintain a fluid, steady stride and a straight, erect posture (Fig. 5.13).

To form a circle while you walk, the foot close to the center of the circle should move straight forward and the outer foot should swing slightly toward the left. Thus a circular track will be formed after a number of steps (Fig. 5.14). This form can be practiced as a moving or static stance.

Third Step: Full Practice (Green Dragon Shows Claw)

The full-practice mud-wading steps combine the footwork with body twisting, arm waving, and palm changes. It appears in the most frequently applied techniques in Bagua and has powerful practical values.

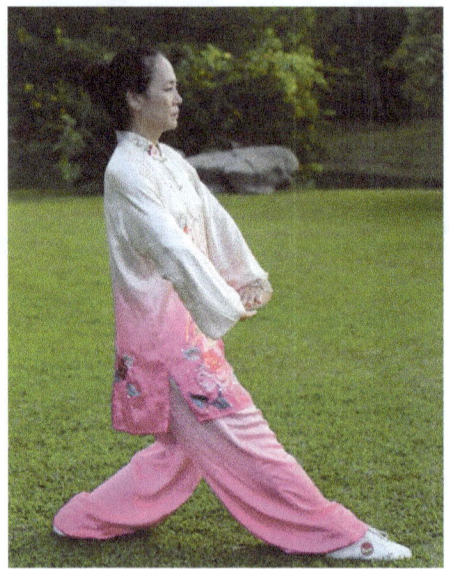

Fig. 5.13. Take the second step forward.

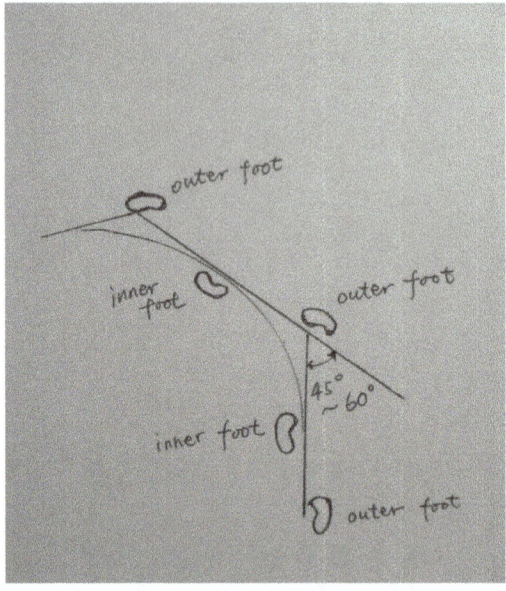

Fig. 5.14. Position of the feet at the inner and outer side.

The difficult part of this form involves the coordination of upper and lower body movements. Over time, the practice of the form, Green Dragon Shows Claw, will enable the learner to have a clear sense of the space and distance, as well as the ability to coordinate all the complicated movements and appreciate the beauty of change of all parts of the body.

1. Continue from the last form of the push-downward palms (Fig. 5.15). Then take the first step forward (Fig. 5.16).

2. Roll the arms upward, making sure the hands stay at the waist. While the left foot steps forward, the two palms turn and face up. Fold the arms and lift the elbows, stopping the palms facing up at the waist (Fig. 5.17).

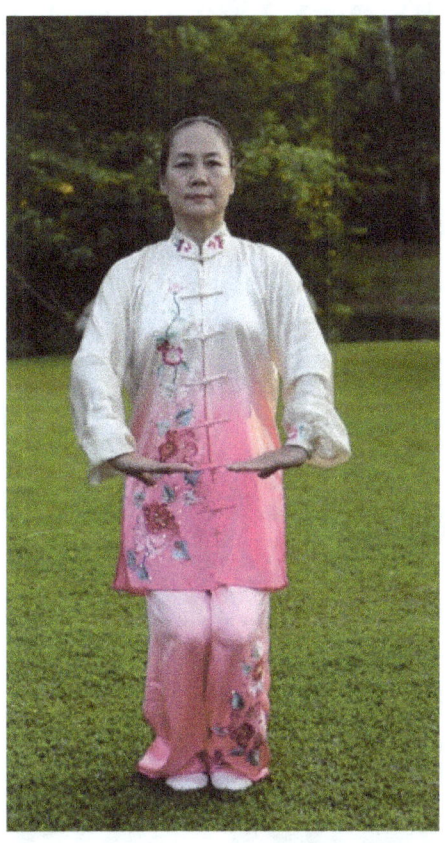

Fig. 5.15. Push palms downward.

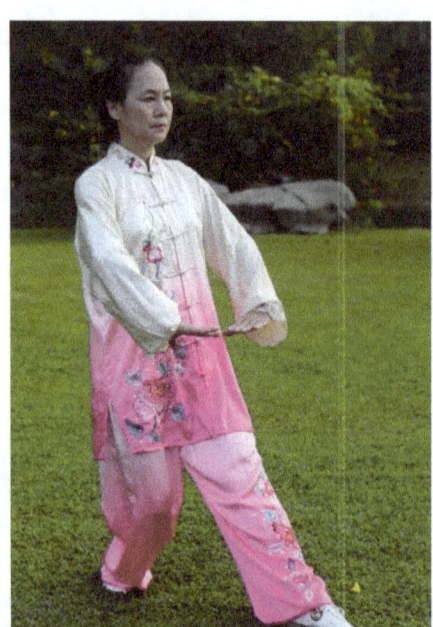

Fig. 5.16. Take the first step forward.

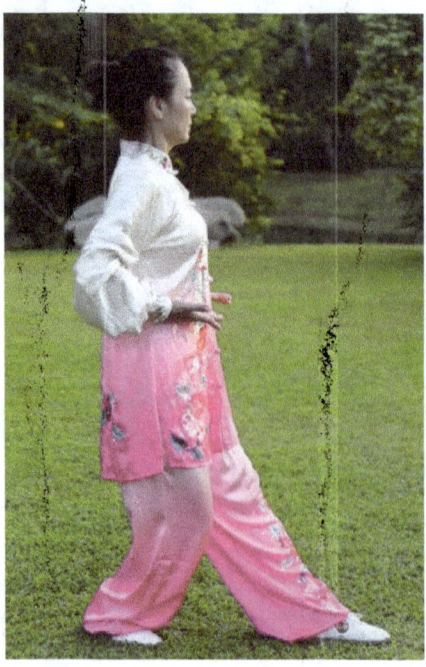

Fig. 5.17. Turn hands up at the waist.

3. Mud-wading with a left arc

Step forward with the right foot, tilting to the left. At the same time, thrust the two palms toward the upper left side, with the palms facing up. The right palm touches the upper part of the left arm near the elbow (Fig. 5.18).

Step forward with the left foot. At the same time, roll the two palms inward and move to the left in an arc. Move the right hand down along the left arm. Keep the left arm raised at the left side of the body, slightly bent, with the wrist cocked and the left palm raised as high as the eyebrow, palm facing left. All fingers of the right palm are separated and pointing upward, except the thumb, which points to the upper right and forms a wide angle with the index finger. The index finger should be kept straight upright while the other fingers are slightly curved.

Sink the right palm behind the left elbow, with the right index finger pointing toward the left elbow. Gaze toward the direction of the left index finger.

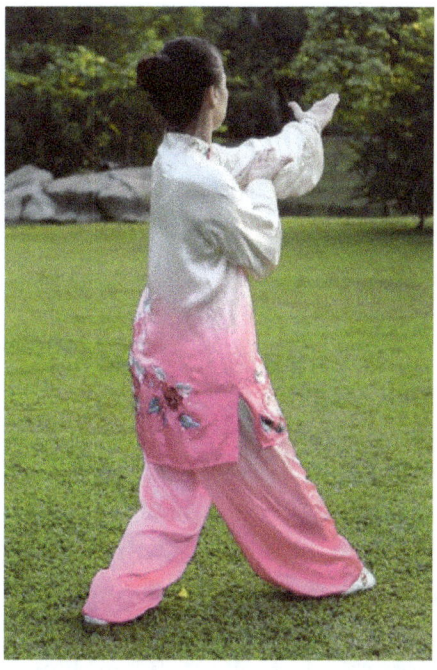

Fig. 5.18. Thrust palms toward upper left.

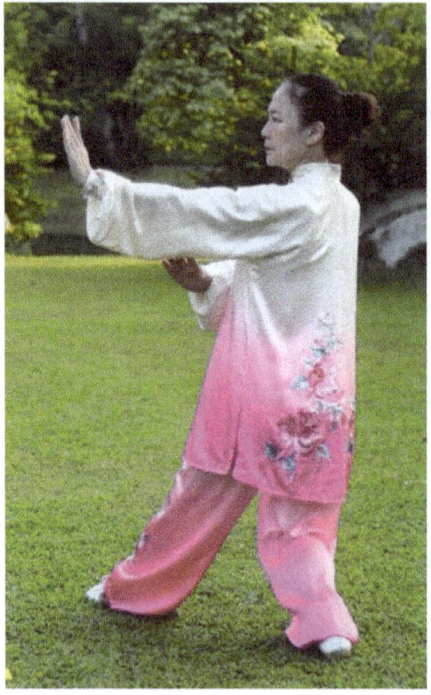

Fig. 5.19.   Green Dragon Shows Claw.

4. Final stance

Wade forward with the left foot, twisting the upper body toward the left as much as possible while raising the arms. Now the most typical form of Bagua, the final form of Green Dragon Shows Claw, is presented flawlessly (Fig. 5.19).

Key Points

1. Keep the neck upright in the whole process, without tilting forward, backward, left, or right.
2. The lower back side should be vertical with a subtle feeling of having the anal sphincter shrunk inward as if withstanding passing a stool. The shoulders should be relaxed and the elbows sunk toward the ground. Feel the *Qi* filling the lower abdomen and make it stuffed and, at the same time, the chest should feel empty and loosened.
3. The wading process should be both swift and steady. The landing of the foot should be light and assured.

5. Fold up

The right foot comes close to the left foot, with the arms stretched to the sides and palms facing upward (Fig. 5.20). Fold the arms, stopping when the hands are above the head, and squat slightly (Fig 5.21).

Push down the palms and stand up at the same time (Fig. 5.22). Let the arms hang loose beside the body, and the folding form is done (Fig. 5.23).

Bagua Palm is a systematic but traditional inner martial arts. The mud-wading steps constitute the most fundamental practice, which has important applications on both fighting and wellness cultivation.

The mud-wading steps are built on walking in a circle with left and right turnings and shifting of the palms. The basic requirements are as follows: twist the head, arm, and waist all toward one side, with the upper body upright and the neck straight as if carrying something on the head, as in the *Ding* from Chapter 4 (Fig. 4.5), withdrawing the chin and maintain inner awareness. Sink the *Qi* (mentally) into the lower belly so that the belly feels solid and the chest feels empty. Sink the hipbones and loosen the waist, lift up the perineum area and slope the hip vertically, and sink the shoulders with the tips of the elbows pointing down to the ground. With the *Qi* staying at the *Dan Tian* (lower belly) area, the body naturally feels like it is sitting vertically on the legs.

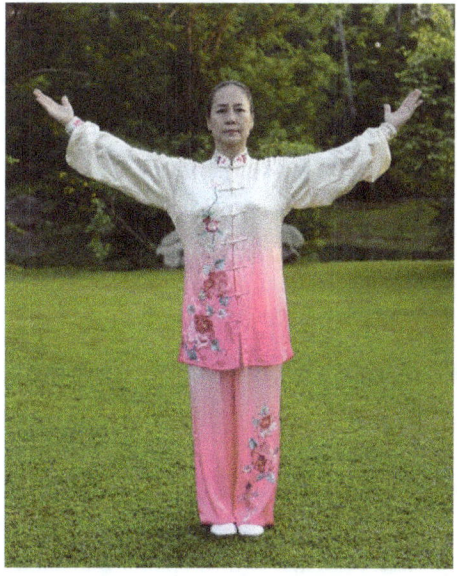

Fig. 5.20. Stretch out.

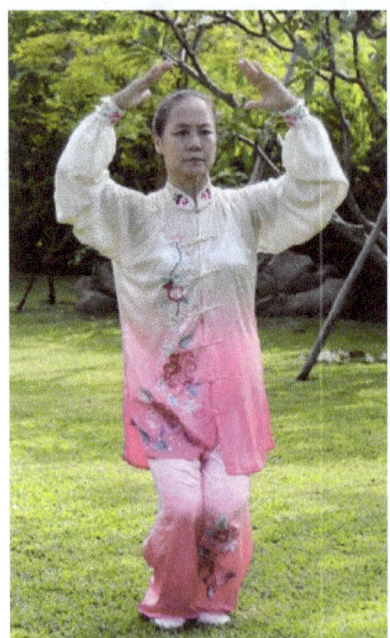

Fig. 5.21. Fold the arms.

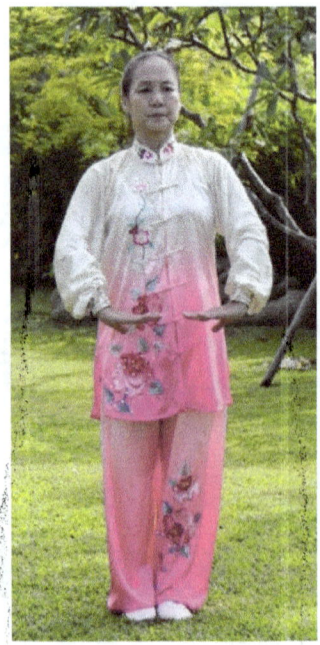

Fig. 5.22. Push down the palms and stand up.

The Mud-Wading Steps 97

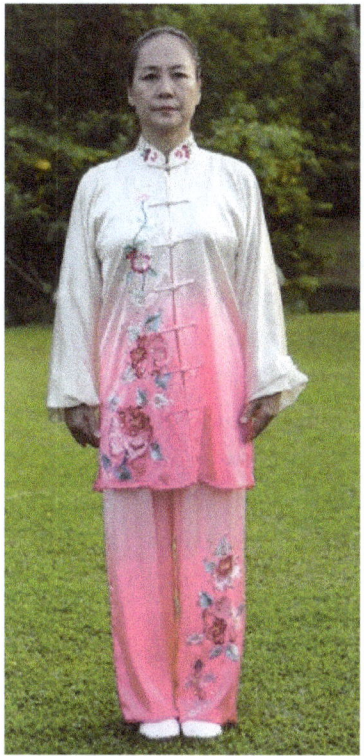

Fig. 5.23. Stand still.

Next, choose a level of height for the center of gravity, be it upper, mid, or lower, and wade through, maintaining the same body height. During the circular walking, the foot should be lifted up and set forward gently, walking like a cat along the circular line. Keep the two legs close to the central line while walking, protecting the crotch area from potential attacks. The two legs should cross each other like a pair of scissors while moving ahead. The back leg, which carries the body weight most of the time, should push off like a punting pole.

Maintain the same height of the body while moving in a circle, with the outswing and inward-latching steps. Be careful, like wading in a muddy area or walking on thin ice.

Beginners or the elderly may start from stances of upper or mid height.

As a typical inner martial art, it takes time to align the body and soul to cultivate the wellness. The rules for the forms should be carefully followed from the beginning, or you may risk drifting farther and farther from the right path.

Each of the rules serves a specific purpose. For example, to keep the neck straight is a requirement to make practitioners more alert and make it easier for them to coordinate the movement of different parts of the body, as well as not to block the flow of the *Qi* around the body. To lift up the perineum area and slope the hip vertically is to facilitate the movements of the lower body and stop the *Qi* from leaking out. To sink the shoulders with the tips of the elbows pointing down to the ground enables the *Qi* to flow to the elbow and the *Jing* to reach the arms and hands for more effective defending and attacking. Sinking the hipbones and loosening the waist will make the belly feel solid and the chest feel empty, and the *Qi* will stay in the *Dan Tian* (lower belly) area. Thus, the practitioner will feel very energetic in the long run.

The waist and hipbone is the pivot connecting the upper and lower body. Only when these parts are relaxed, can the *Qi* from *Dan Tian* be able to reach the legs and feet.

To perform wading with bent legs while lifting up the center of the foot, the toes must hold onto the ground. This will make the landing of the foot stable and powerful like what happens when a tiger walks. It was said that grasping the ground with the five toes of the foot like a root creates a momentum powerful enough to shake the mountains, as believed to be shown by the tiger.

Besides the surging steps, there is another type with a shorter step called *Chui* (捶droopy) step. It is almost the same as the surging step except it does not require extra forward surging before the front foot lands. In Weaving Stance Bagua, it can be used to connect the outward-turning or inward-latching steps. When there is body turning, the droopy step is more suitable as it enables faster turning with shorter steps.

A thousand miles begin with a single step. With perfectly tuned wading steps, you will be fully ready for the magnificent world of Bagua.

Appendix

A more abstract example is the superposition of waves with different frequencies. The four waves from the top add together to form the final actual wave at the bottom. The first wave, with the lowest frequency, decides the final general frequency (Fig. 5.24).

As shown in Chapter 3, the superposition of vectors F1 and F2 forms F.

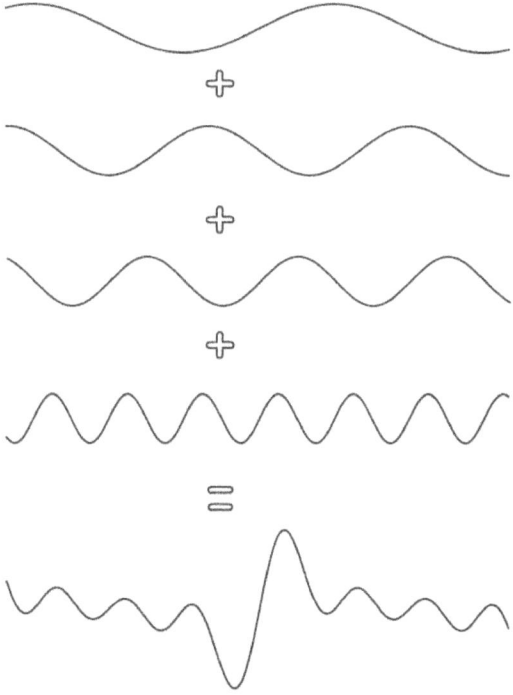

Fig. 5.24. The superposition of waves with different frequencies.

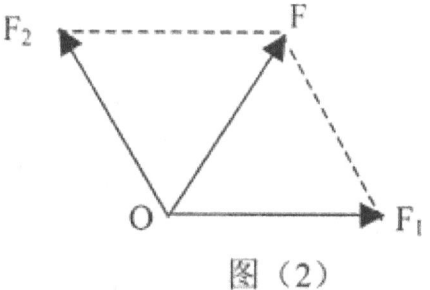

图 (2)

Fig. 5.25. The superposition of vectors.

6
The New 64 Forms of Weaving Stance Bagua Palm

Brief Introduction

The forms of Bagua introduced in this book are the forms practiced by Master Ge Chun Yan, who has been the National Champion of Bagua in China for five years, a record unbroken. Due to the elegant interpretation of the forms, Master Li Jun Feng and Master Ge Chun Yan together made Bagua Palm shine in the very first mainland China *gongfu* movie *Deadly Fury*, which was made in 1983 and won the Award of National Movie Excellence.

The forms of Bagua were originally spread out from Beijing, and this particular 64 forms for this book consolidated the forms practiced by Master Sun Zhi Jun and Liu Jing Ru from Beijing, and Master Sha Guo Zheng from Yunnan.

A good set of martial art forms must come with scientific and reasonable training methods. Based on the training tradition of the official Martial Arts Team of Beijing, and under the instruction of the Bagua Palm masters, we firstly focused on the repetitive training of the Bagua fundamentals and basic forms, such as *Tang Ni* (mud-wading) Steps and *Bai* (摆swing) *Kou* (扣latch) steps, the twisting, wrapping, drilling and turning of the body movements, etc.

On top of that, we have placed great emphasis on the rhythm and style of the performance. Thus, whoever learns this form should pay particular attention to the fundamentals and the rhythm of the practice and performance. By working both hard and smart, the trainee should make this particular style of Bagua stand out, which means to be complete with the spirit of three animals: to move like a swimming dragon, to change forms like an eagle wheeling in the air, and to turn like a swift monkey. All the movements should be light but not rootless, steady but not stuck, soft but not loose. During the practice of the forms, we should do it with strength and yet grace, be flexible and yet vigorous, move steadily with clear cut *Bai* (摆swing) and *Kou* (扣latch) steps, keeping focused from beginning to end, connecting all the forms well, and finishing them as one single form.

List of the 64 Forms

Starting form
1. Sink palm
2. Left push palm
3. Inward-latching step with shielding elbow
4. Crouch step with forward-lifting palm
5. Step forward with swaying palms
6. Smashing palm with a left turn
7. Left and right blocking palm
8. Smashing palm with a right turn
9. Inward-latching left slipping palm
10. Right push palm
11. Inward-latching step with shielding elbow
12. Right stealthy tuck-in backward palm
13. Forward-step piercing palm
14. Right-turn cover palm
15. Stride and tuck-in striking palm
16. Turn with whirling arms
17. Back-hand thump
18. Cloud hand right tuck-in palm
19. Turning cloud palm
20. Squat hugging palm
21. Piercing palm with left knee lifted
22. Forward right thrust palm
23. Turn to thrust palm left and right
24. Backward-leaning plane turning palm
25. Withdraw step tuck-in palm
26. Forward-step piercing palm
27. Turn for wiping palm
28. Hugging palms to roll
29. Withdraw-step diverting palm

30. Forward-step pressing palm
31. Paring and wiping palm
32. Side thrusting palm
33. Forward-chopping palm
34. Front cross-step chopping palm
35. Open stance rightward paring palm
36. Inward-latching step rotate body
37. Lean back kick with double thrusting palm
38. Crouching stance piercing palm
39. Heaven drilling palm with side-by-side foot stance
40. Tuck-in and left-and-right bumping palm
41. Outward swing and inward-latching steps and cloudy palm
42. Horizontal opening chop with a turn
43. Left stride tuck-in and bumping palm
44. Join up and tuck in leftward opening palm
45. Right drilling palm
46. Windmill-style chopping palm
47. Lifting and bumping palm
48. Right wiping palm
49. Left wiping palm
50. Right tuck-in palm
51. Left wiping palm
52. Right wiping palm
53. Left tuck-in palm
54. Joint holding palms
55. Turn with drilling palms
56. Holding up palms
57. Joint holding palms
58. Left heaven drilling palm
59. Horizontal pushing palm
60. Open stance up pushing palm
61. Hugging palm with folded body
62. Double-pressing palm after a turn
63. Right piercing palm with inward-latching step
64. Left push palm
Closing form

Starting form

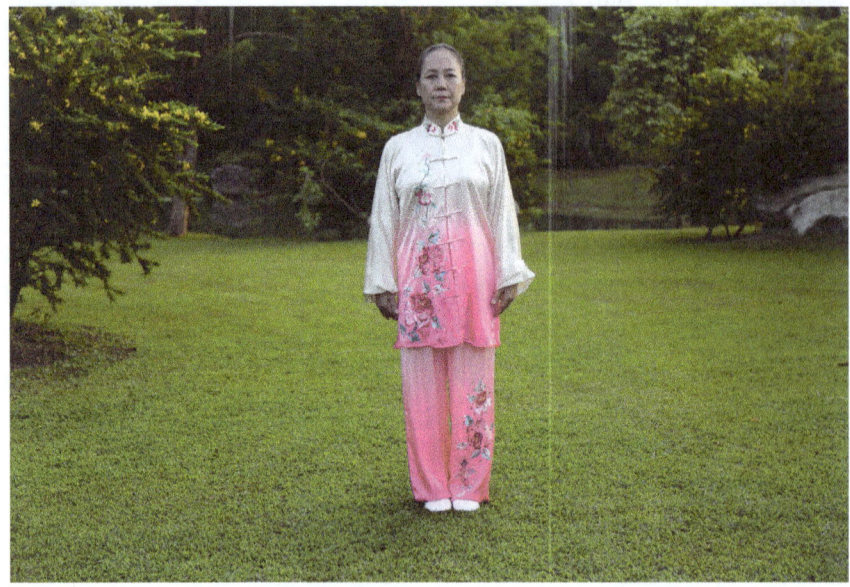

Fig. 6.1.

Preparatory Posture

Face south and stand with the feet close to each other, keeping the legs naturally straight, arms hanging at the side, palms relaxed and facing inward naturally. Keep the upper body, including the head and neck, upright, the chest and abdomen relaxed, shoulders hanging down loosely, mouth closed while breathing naturally, eyes gazing level. At the same time, leave all the trivialities in daily life behind. Just relax and feel the *Qi* and blood running inside the whole body. Feel connected with nature and merge yourself with heaven and earth, dancing with *Yin* and *Yang*, and feel their beauty (Fig. 6.1).

Starting Form: The Sink Palm

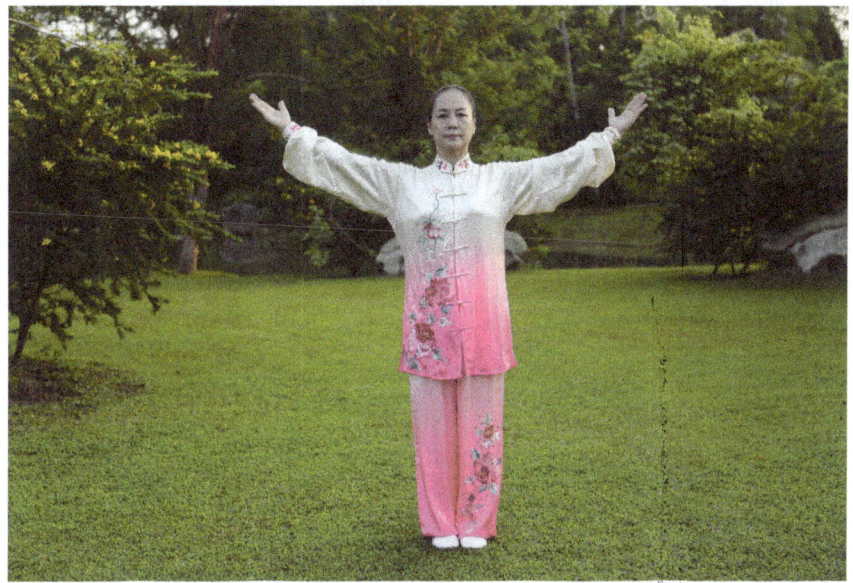

Fig. 6.2.

1. Raise both arms from the side of the body, turn the forearms while moving upwards and make the palms facing upwards, fingers naturally separated (Fig. 6.2).

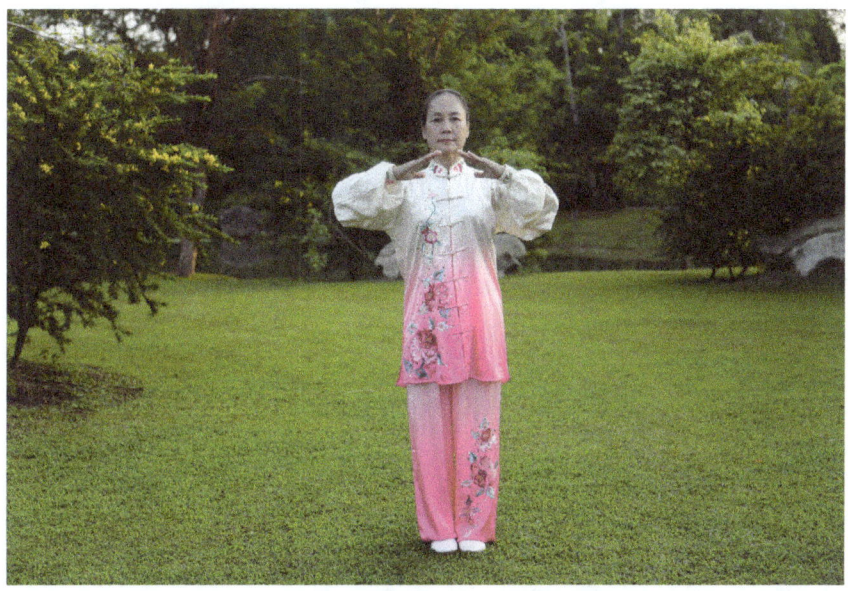

Fig. 6.3.

2. Next, fold the forearms around the elbow until the palms face down and be prepared to push downwards once the knees start to bend (Fig. 6.3). While squatting down slowly, push both palms downward until they reach the front of the lower abdomen, arms curved and upper body straight (Fig. 6.4).

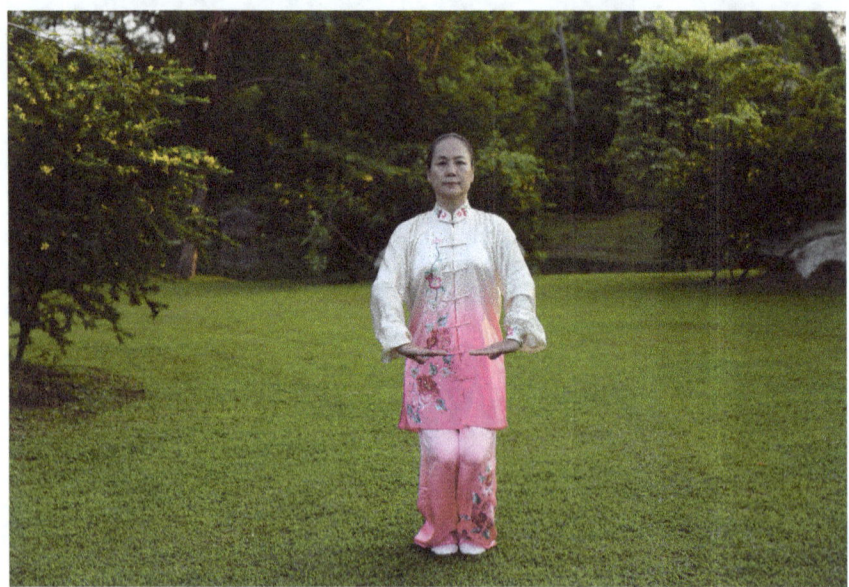

Fig. 6.4.

Key Points

1. Inhale while raising the arms, and exhale while pushing the hands downward.
2. Imagine absorbing the *Qi* from the universe and merging it into your body; feel energized and confident.
3. Squat and push the hands downward concurrently from start to finish.

The New 64 Forms of Weaving Stance Bagua Palm   107

1. Sink palm

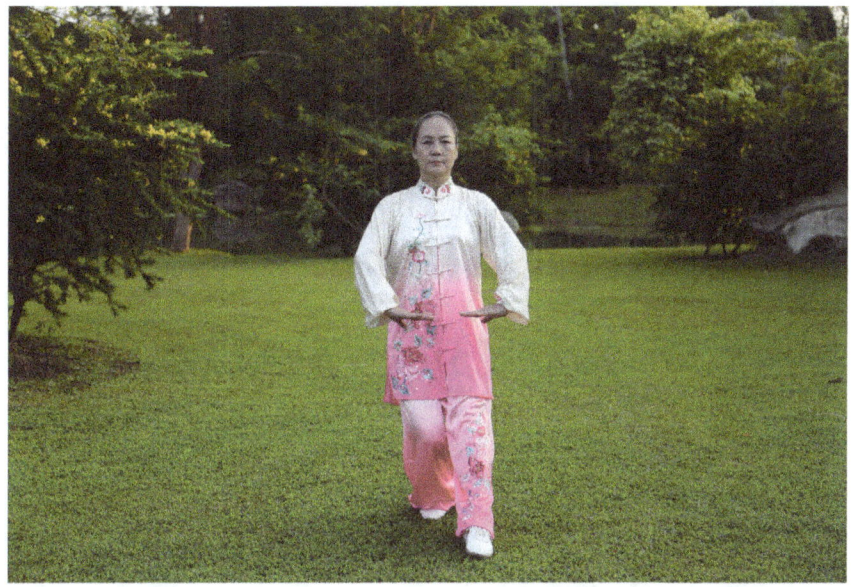

Fig. 6.5.

1. Keep the posture and start the mud-wading steps. Lift the left leg slowly while the right leg stays bent, then move the left foot forward slowly with the sole parallel to the ground, and the center of gravity of the body starts to move forward (Fig.6.5).

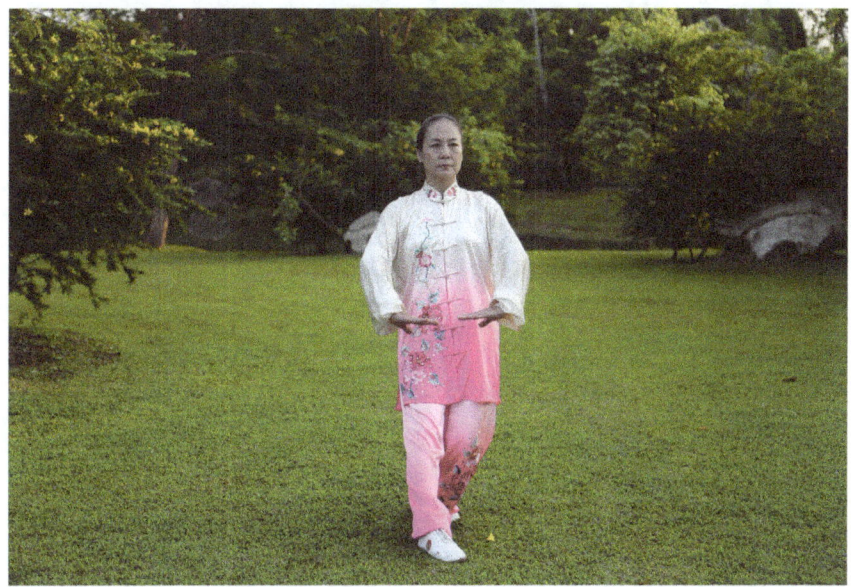

Fig. 6.6.

2. While moving forward, the right leg should push backward forcefully against the ground, giving the left foot engergy to move further along the ground to form a big step. Once the left foot lands, the right foot should start to move forward in the same manner with the thigh pulling the calf, swinging forward and leveraging on its inertia. The inner sides of the knees will rub against each other slightly while moving forward with the sole parallel and close to the ground. Upon landing, the right foot points slightly inwards (toward the center of the circle) (Fig. 6.6).

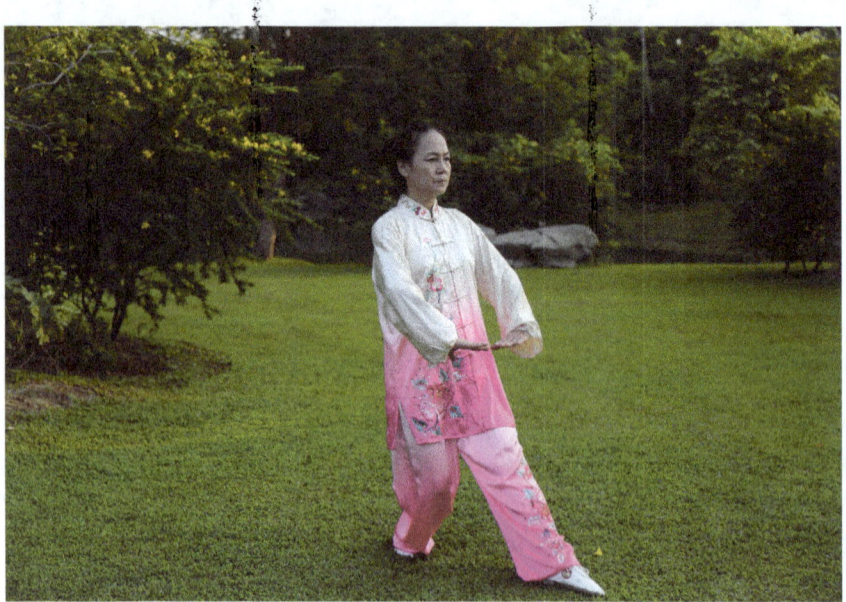

Fig. 6.7.

3. Keep moving forward, with the left leg pushing backward forcefully against the ground, giving the right foot energy to move further along the ground to form a big step. When the right foot has landed, move the left foot forward in the direction the right foot points (southeast). Other requirements stay the same (Fig. 6.7).

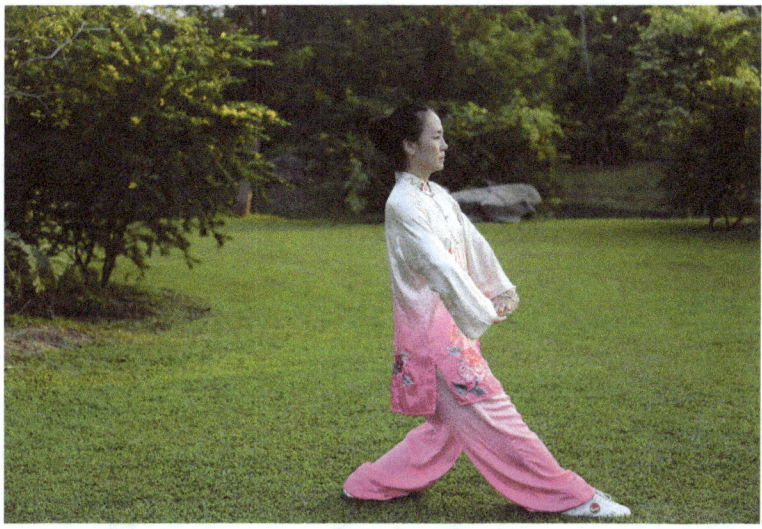

Fig. 6.8.

4. While moving forward, the right leg should push backward forcefully against the ground, enabling the left foot to move forward in a big step along the ground. Next, the right foot should move forward for the fourth step, while the foot points slightly inward toward the east upon landing (Fig. 6.8).

Key Points

1. Move forward and form an arc toward the left side with the initial four steps. From the very first left step forward, the movement should be slow but powerful, symbolizing a starting of the action with inner force. Next, continue with the mud-wading steps at a pace suitable for each individual. Keep the soles parallel to the ground as much as possible while lifting and landing the feet. Once the front foot has landed, bend the knee simultaneously and maintain the height of the posture to avoid any up-and-down motion. The two legs need to be so close to each other that they rub slightly while crossing each other. The two knees need to stay relatively close. The front foot should move swiftly without lifting too high from the ground. The body weight should stay on the back leg. When the front foot wades forward as if through mud, the back leg should push against the ground forcefully, adding to the momentum of the forward movement to increase the pace.

2. While the legs are moving with power, the abdomen needs to be relaxed so as to allow the *Qi* to flow smoothly around. The arms should be kept steady in front of the abdomen with the thumb and forefingers wide apart to form an arc.
3. While moving, gaze forward with a sparkle in the eyes to match the strong inner forward momentum.

2. Left push palm

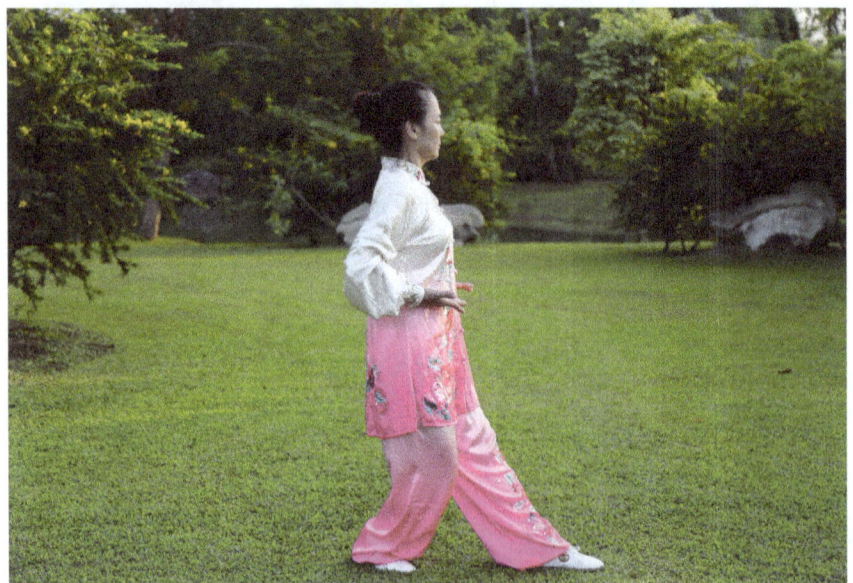

Fig. 6.9.

1. Keep moving forward, the left leg pushing backward against the ground and the right foot moving forward. When the right foot has landed, move the left foot forward for the fifth step. At the same time, turn the arms and withdraw the elbows, placing the palms beside the waist, palms facing up (Fig. 6.9).

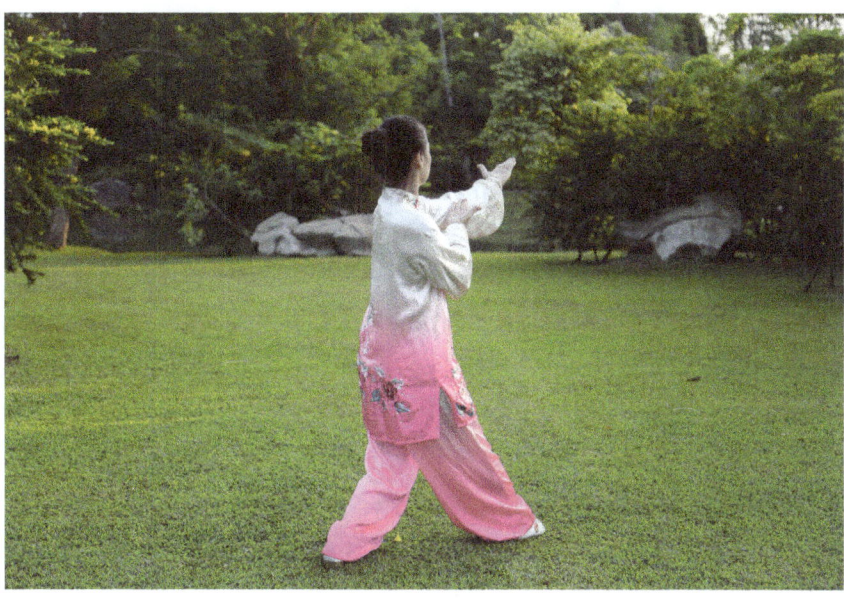

Fig. 6.10.

2. Keep the mud-wading arc toward the left and place the right foot forward for the sixth step, pointing northeast upon landing. At the same time, both palms should thrust forward to the upper left, with the palms still facing up and the back side of the right palm touching the left arm on top of the elbow joint (Fig. 6.10).

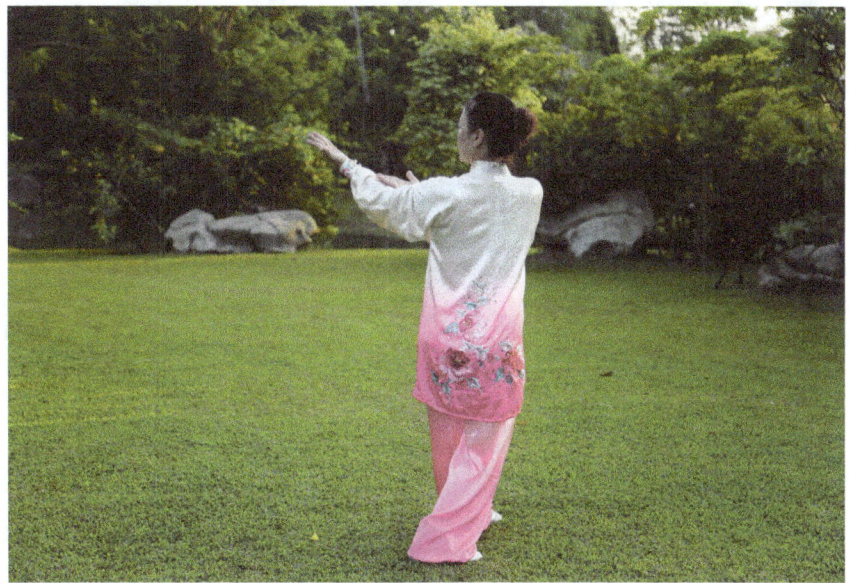

Fig. 6.11.

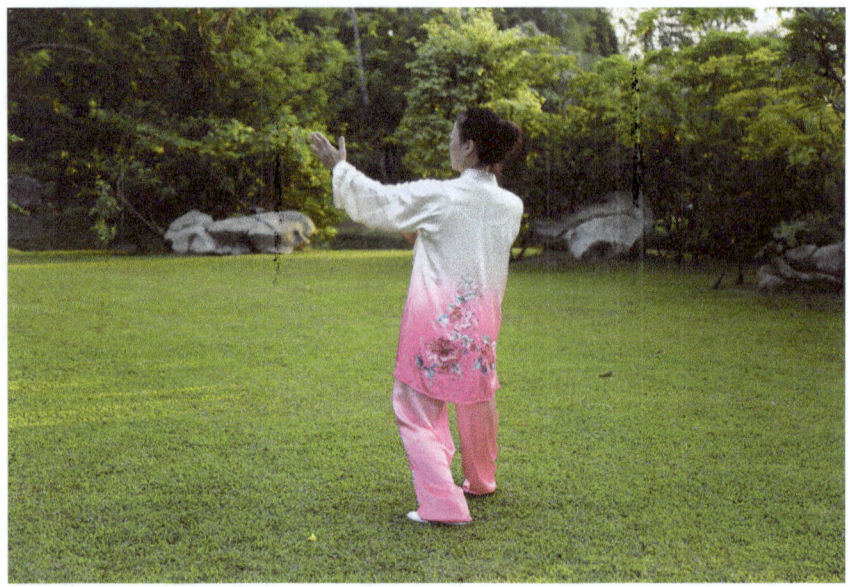

Fig. 6.12.

3. The left foot should move forward for the seventh step, and right foot for the eighth step, with the front foot pointing north. At the same time, roll both palms inward and move to the left in an arc. The right hand should move down along the left arm (Figs. 6.11 and 6.12).

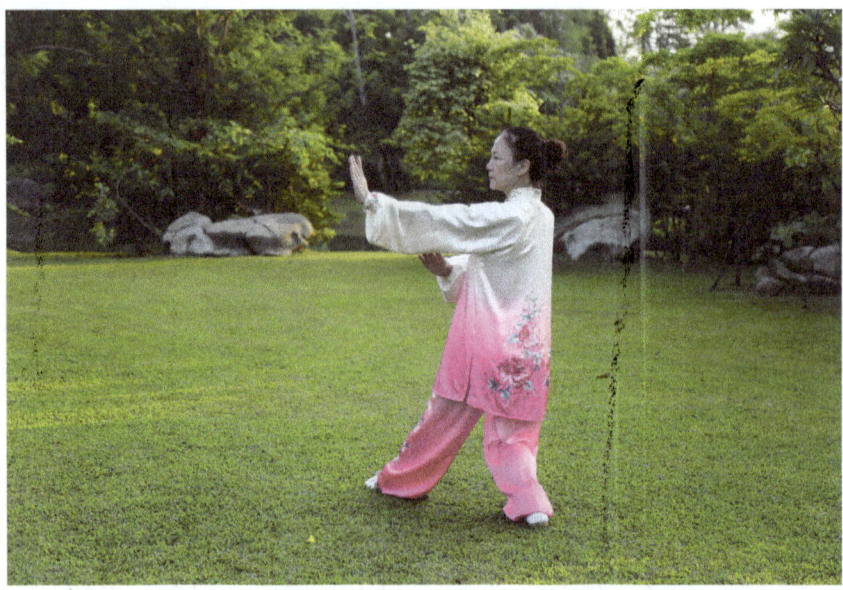

Fig. 6.13.

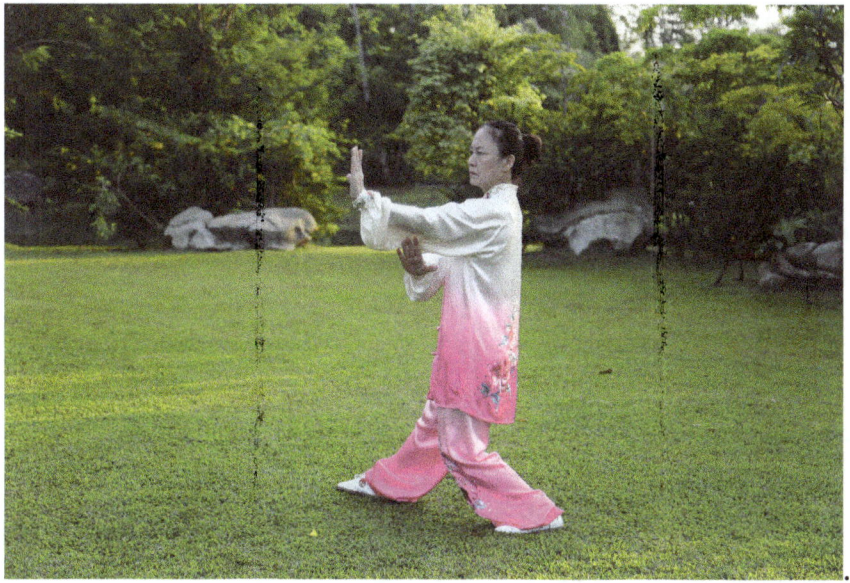

Fig. 6.14.

4. The left foot should move forward for the ninth step, and the right foot for the 10th step, with the front foot pointing to the west, the left arm raised and slightly bent at the left side of the body, the wrist cocked, and the left palm raised as high as the eyebrow, palm facing left. All fingers of the left palm should be separated and pointed upward, except the thumb, which should point to the upper right and form a wide angle with the index finger. The index finger should be held straight upright while the other fingers are slightly curved.

   The right palm should sink behind the left elbow, with the right index finger directed toward the left elbow. Gaze toward the direction of the left index finger (Figs. 6.13 and 6.14).

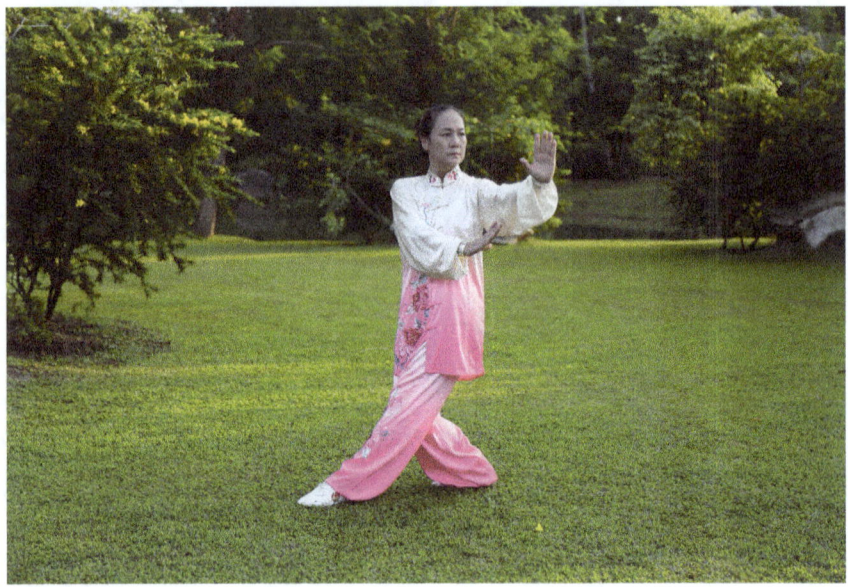

Fig. 6.15.

4. The left foot wades forward for the 11th step, and the upper body twists toward the left together with the raised arms as much as possible. The whole body now is back to the starting point (Fig. 6.15).

Key Points

1. Keep the neck upright in the whole process, without tilting forward, backward, left, or right.
2. The lower back side should be vertical with a subtle feeling of having the anal sphincter shrunk inward as if withholding a stool. The shoulders should be relaxed and the elbows sunk toward the ground. Feel the Qi fill the lower abdomen, making it stuffed, and at the same time, the chest feels empty and loose.
3. The wading process should be both swift and steady. The landing of the foot should be light and assured.
4. The beginning of the forms is always extremely important, as it sets the foundation for the whole practice. The initial two forms, sink palm and left push palm, are the very basic forms of Bagua Palm. Solid leg work and basic skills, as well as the inner feeling and momentum, should be observed with great care.

These 11 steps are suitable for martial art competitions, where the practice area tends to be bigger. For the daily practice of ordinary people, the number of steps can be adjusted accordingly to adapt for the smaller practice area with smaller circles.

3. Inward-latching step with shielding elbow

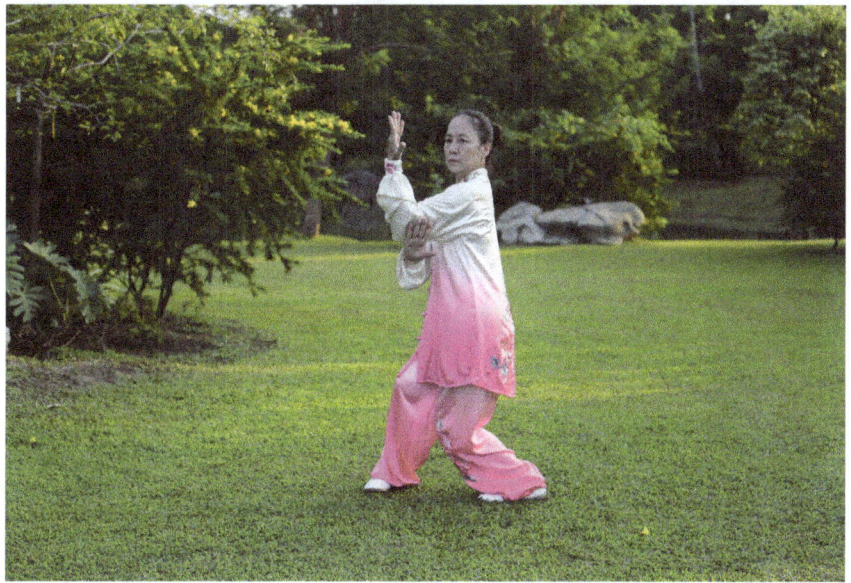

Fig. 6.16.

Follow the last form, with the right foot moving just past the left toe with an inward-latching step. The distance between the two feet should be 10–20 cm, with the heels propped outward and the two feet directly perpendicular to each other. The knees should stay close, with the left side of right knee touching the left knee, the left hip turned inward to twist left. At the same time, the left forearm should turn clockwise and move to the right with the elbow folded until touching the chest, with the left palm facing left. The back side of the right palm should touch the outside of the left upper arm. The upper body should turn toward the right as much as possible (Fig. 6.16).

4. Crouch step with forward-lifting palm

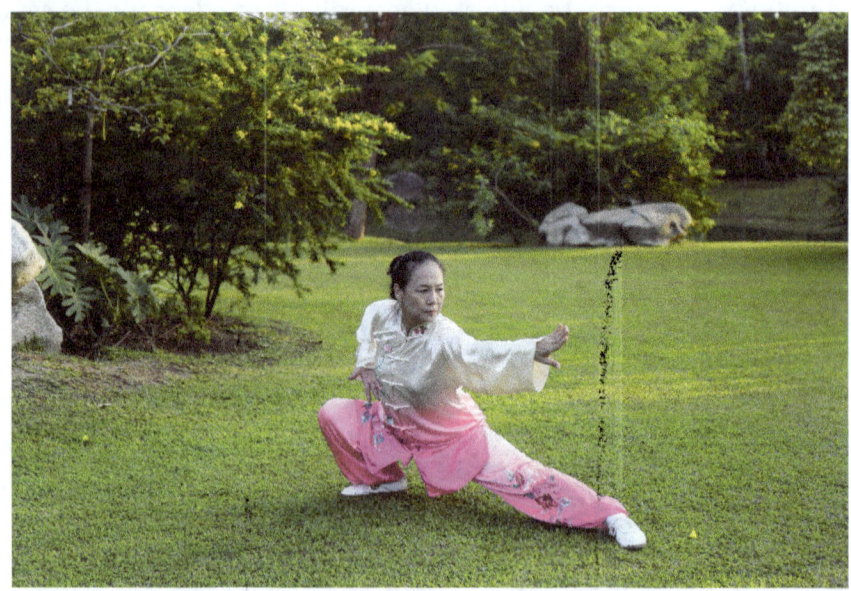

Fig. 6.17.

Bend the right knee outward and squat down fully, quickly stretching out left foot a little toward the southeast direction. The left foot hooks inward slightly with the whole sole touching the ground. The left leg should be stretched straight and stay close to the ground to form the left crouching step. At the same time, turn the left forearm clockwise and wave the left palm, first in a downward arc and then leftward, until the whole left arm is straight and leveled with the shoulder, keeping the wrist straight and palm facing backward. The right hand is folded at the waist, palm facing up, while the whole upper body leans naturally toward the left foot (Fig. 6.17).

5. Step forward with swaying palms

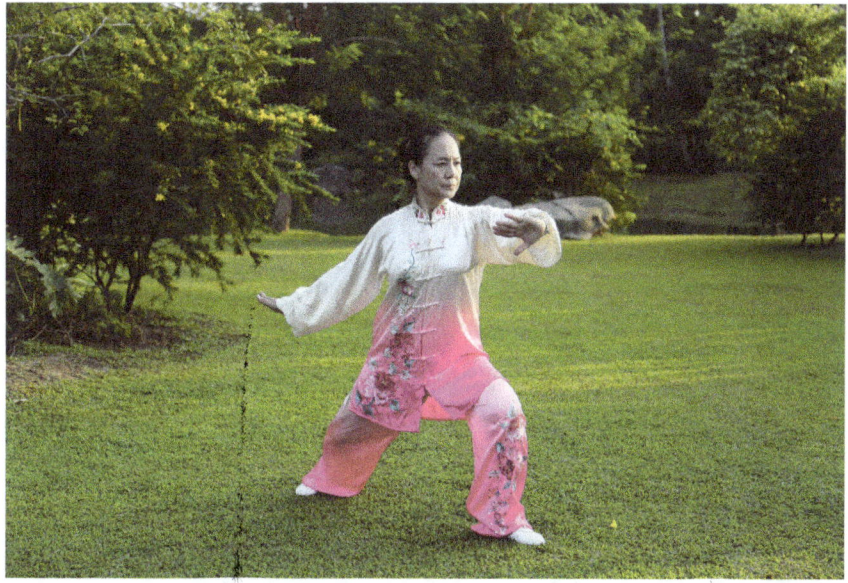

Fig. 6.18.

1. Push off the right leg to lift the body. Bend the left leg and bow forward to move the center of gravity forward. Naturally swing the right arm backward until nearly straight, palm down. The left arm should fold naturally, ready to move forward (Fig. 6.18).

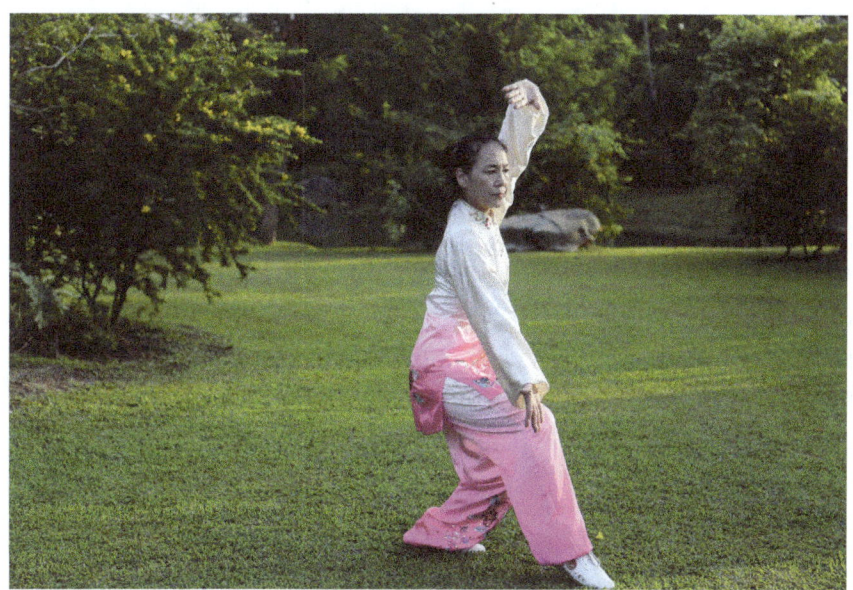

Fig. 6.19.

2. Continue to push off with the right leg, with the body weight moving onto the left leg. Shift the right foot forward (a little in the southeast direction) with the right palm swaying forward along the outside of the right thigh, moving the palm forward until the front side of the knee, keeping the right arm slightly curved. While the left arm bends and forms an elbow block upward, keep the left hand clearly above your head, palms facing up. Bend the legs and gaze forward (Fig. 6.19).

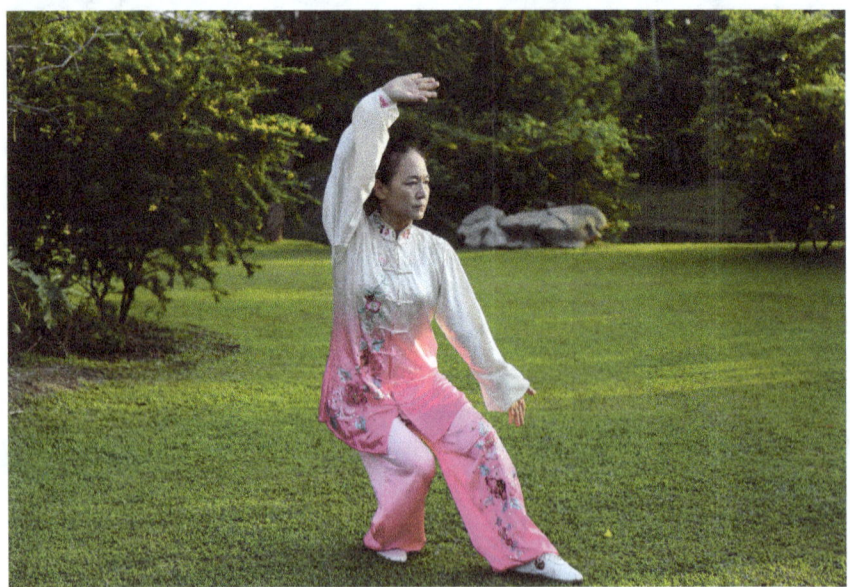

Fig. 6.20.

3. Continue to move the body weight forward, pushing off with the left leg to drive the right foot wading forward. Wave the right hand in an upward arc, bending the right arm and forming an elbow block upward, keeping your hand clearly above your head, palms facing up. At the same time, sway the left palm from above the head backward, downward and then forward in a circle, while the left foot starts to wade forward. Keep swaying the left palm along the outside of the left thigh, moving it forward until the front side of the left knee, keeping the left arm slightly curved while gazing forward (Fig. 6.20).

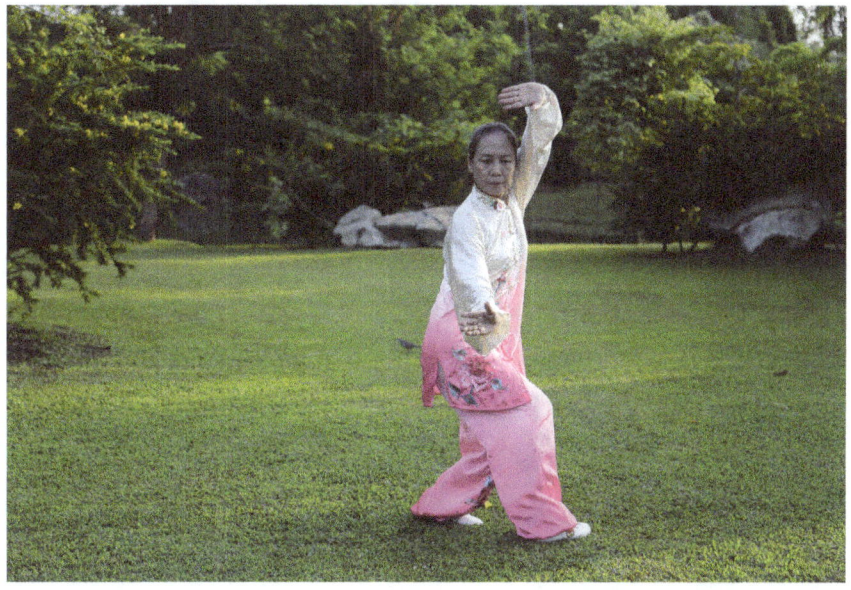

Fig. 6.21.

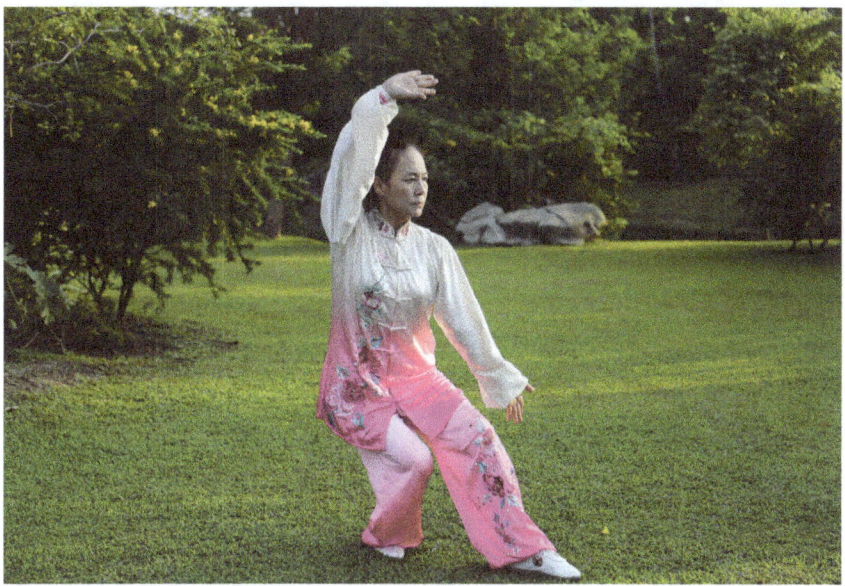

Fig. 6.22.

4. Repeat steps 2–3 (Figs. 6.21 and 6.22). There are a total of four steps in this form.

Key Points

1. When you are capable of mastering the mud-wading steps, move faster to enhance the momentum.
2. The two arms should sway in a circle vertical to the ground with a big radius. The swaying should be coordinated well with the footwork.
3. Reduce the number of steps if space is limited.

6. Smashing palm with a left turn

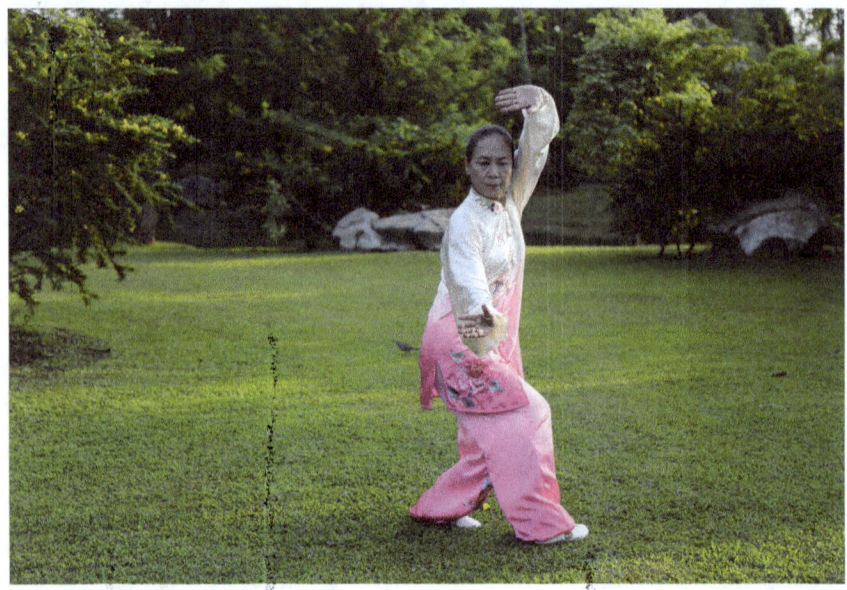

Fig. 6.23.

1. After the left foot has landed, the right foot continues to step forward, landing toward the east or northeast direction, with the right foot latching inward. At the same time, the right palm continues to swing backward, downward to the side of the right hip, palm forward. The left palm should continue to swing forward and upward, and finally form an elbow block upward. Look toward the right hand (Fig. 6.23).

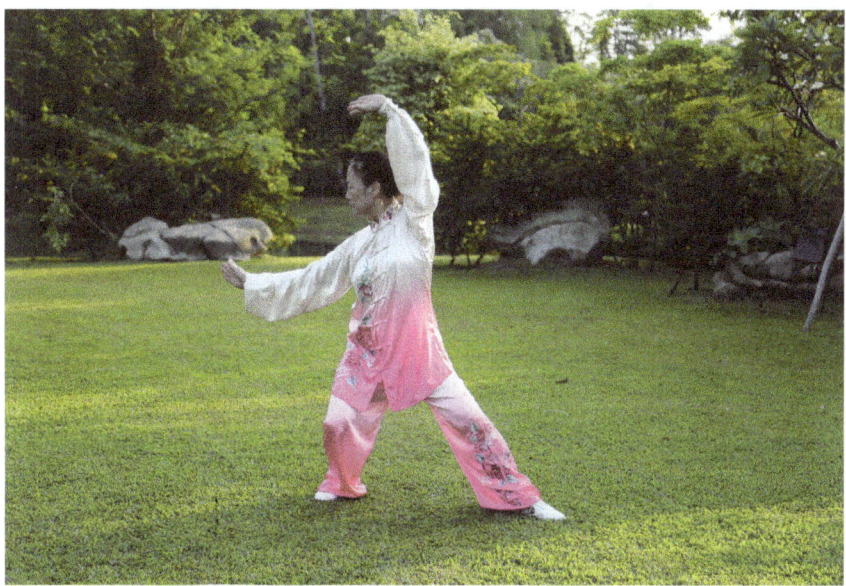

Fig. 6.24.

2. Turn left with the left foot stepping backward toward the left side (southeast direction), both legs squatting with the center of gravity in between the legs but slightly closer to the right. The right hand should be placed behind the body to the right. Look toward the right hand (Fig. 6.24).

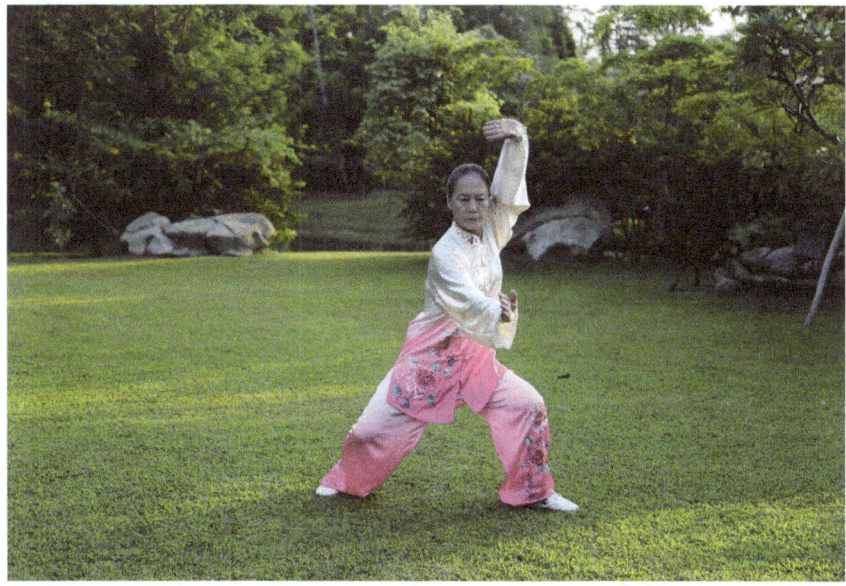

Fig. 6.25.

3. Turn left forcefully, smashing the right palm toward the left. The center of gravity moves slightly leftward, with the left leg bent and the right leg slightly bent. The right elbow should be slightly bent, while the left arm forms an elbow block upward. Look toward the right hand (Fig. 6.25).

7. Left and right blocking palm

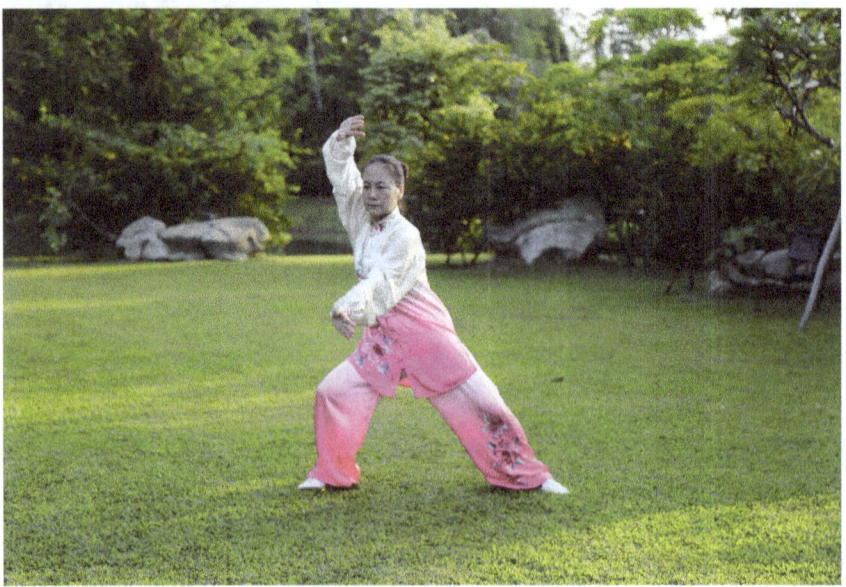

Fig. 6.26.

1. Push off the left leg to move the center of gravity rightward and turn right, leveraging on this momentum, while the right arm swings to the upper right and forms a palm block upward (Fig. 6.26).

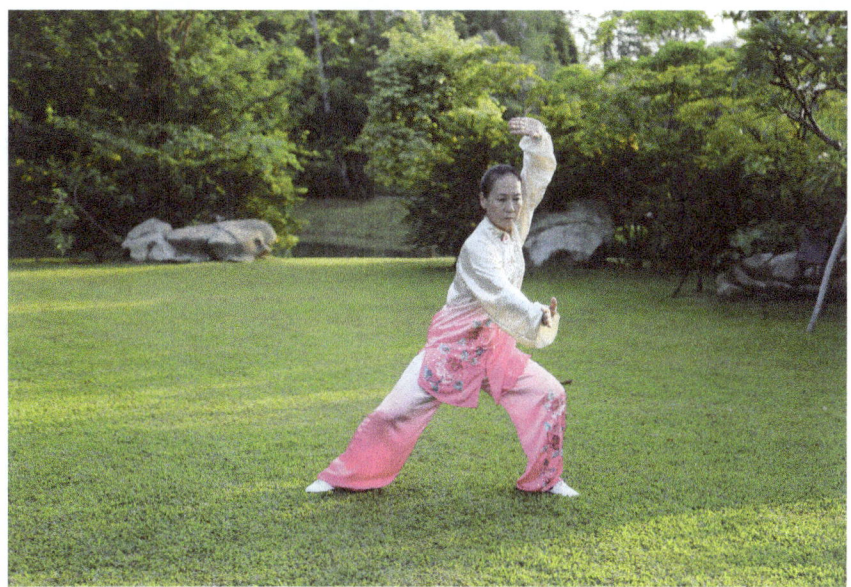

Fig. 6.27.

2. Push off hard with the right leg to move the center of gravity leftward and turn left, leveraging on this momentum, while the left arm swings to the upper left and forms a palm block upward. At the same time, the right palm waves rightward and downward, and then leftward in an arc. Turn the head to the left with the move (Fig. 6.27).

Key Points

The range of body shifting and turning should be wide and accelerated in the process.

8. Smashing palm with a right turn

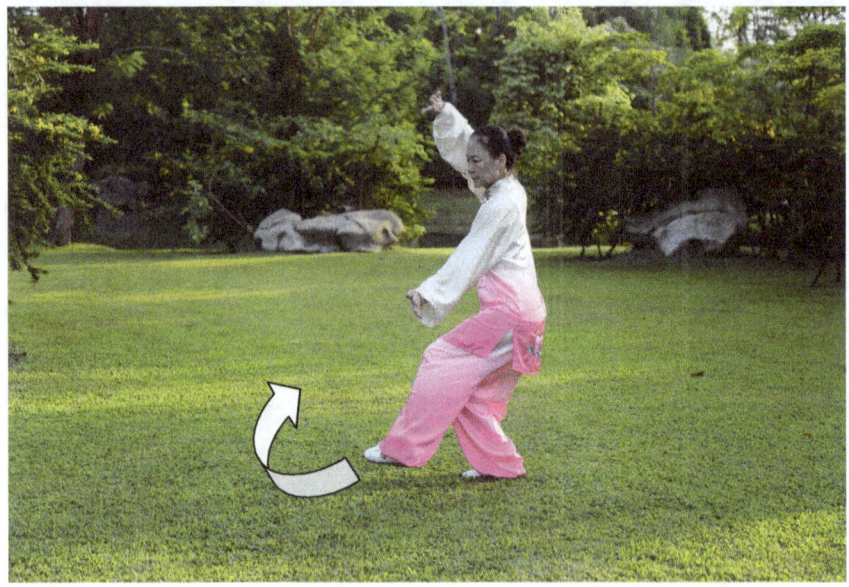

Fig. 6.28.

1. Push off with the left leg to turn right, quickly stepping rightward with the left foot and land toward the west or northwest direction, with the foot latch inward (Fig. 6.28).

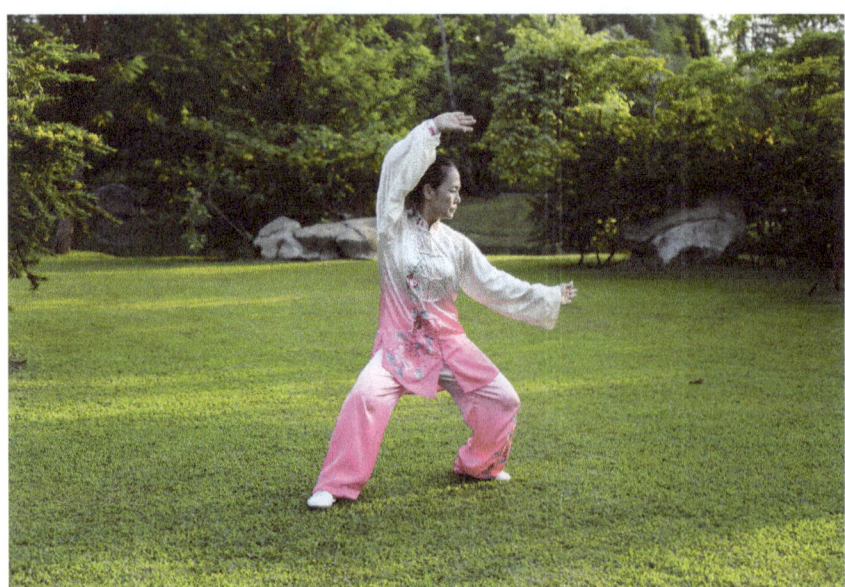

Fig. 6.29.

Turn right and land with the left foot latching inward. Step the right foot backward toward right side (southwest direction), both legs squatting with the center of gravity in between the legs, slightly closer to the left. The left hand is placed behind the body to the left. Look toward the left hand (Fig. 6.29).

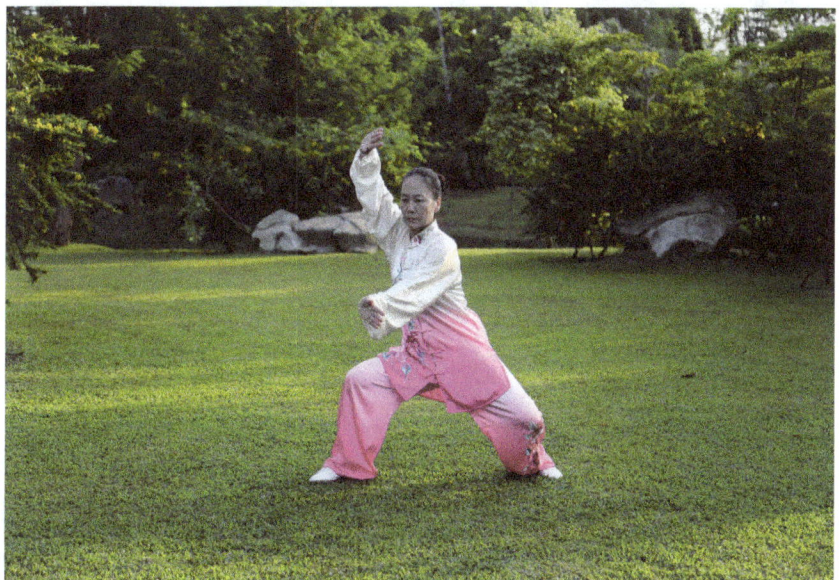

Fig. 6.30.

2. Turn forcefully right, smashing the left palm toward the right. The center of gravity should move slightly rightward, with the right leg bent and the left leg slightly bent. The right arm forms an elbow block upward. Look toward the left hand (Fig. 6.30).

Key Points

1. The whole turning and palm smashing movement need to be smooth. The palm smash out, unified with the momentum of the whole body, not just the force of the arm. The force needs to originate from the leg, controlled by the waist and transferred to the arm.
2. The range of movement shall be wide and followed with speed and power in the process. After the smashing palm, the left leg might have a small step toward the right as an adjustment.

9. Inward-latching left slipping palm

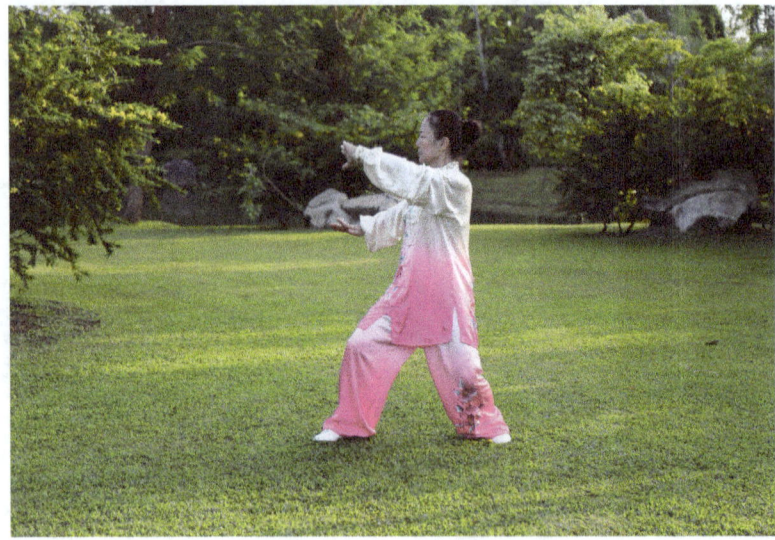

Fig. 6.31a.

1. Turn slightly right, the right palm waving slowly toward the lower right side, palm facing lower right. At the same time, the left palm swings toward the upper right side while the left arm twists clockwise, palm facing down tilted, with the head turned slightly right (Fig. 6.31a). This is the preparation for the next part which should be performed slowly but with potential power.

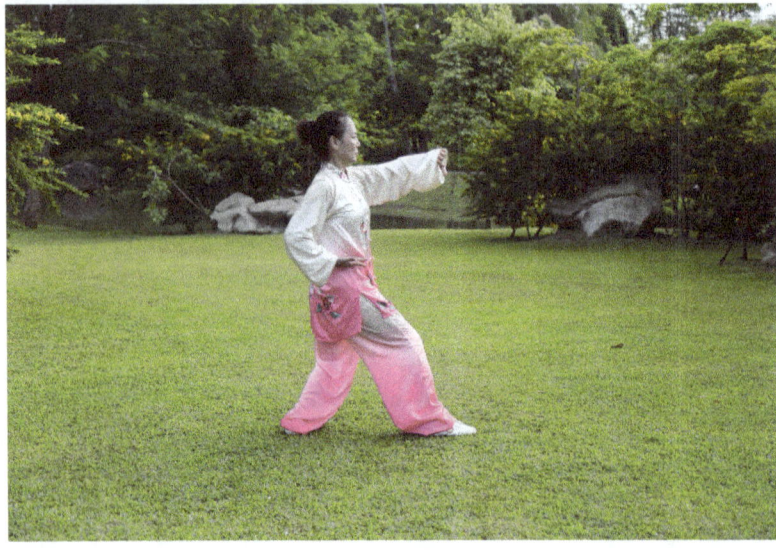

Fig. 6.31b.

2. Turn left quickly with right foot moving swiftly past the left foot with an inward-latching step. At the same time, the left hand waves to the left in an arc with the momentum of the turning, the left arm bent slightly. The right hand turns clockwise until the palm faces up, staying close to the right waist (Fig. 6.31b). After the right foot has landed, the body continues to turn left, with the left arm moving close to the body gradually, keeping the palm facing outside tilted.

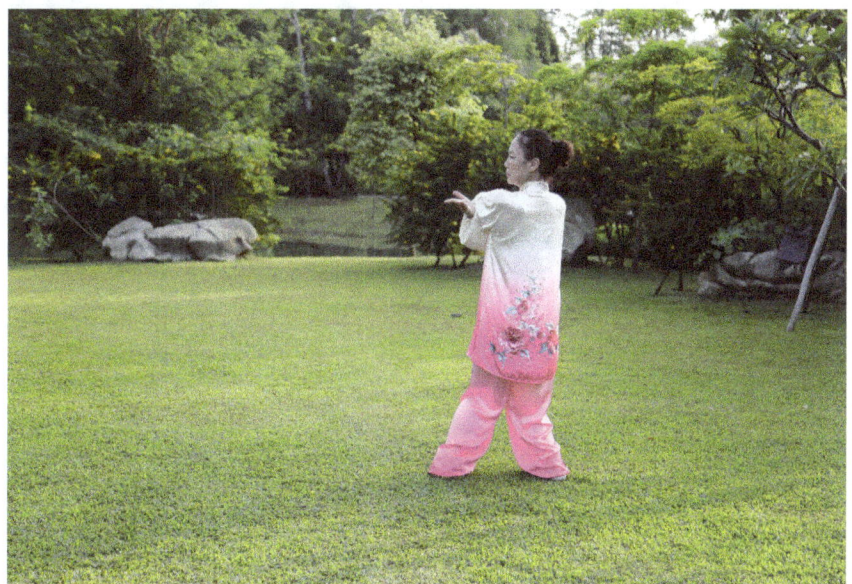

Fig. 6.32.

At the same time, the right palm slightly rubs the body and slips out to the left in front of the chest and the left armpit, palm facing up. Turn the head to the left (Fig. 6.32).

Key Points

1. Turn aggressively in a large angle, turning right and then quickly turning left.
2. The turning of the body should be coordinated with the slipping of the palm. Both should finish at the same time and the whole body should remain twisted.

10. Right push palm

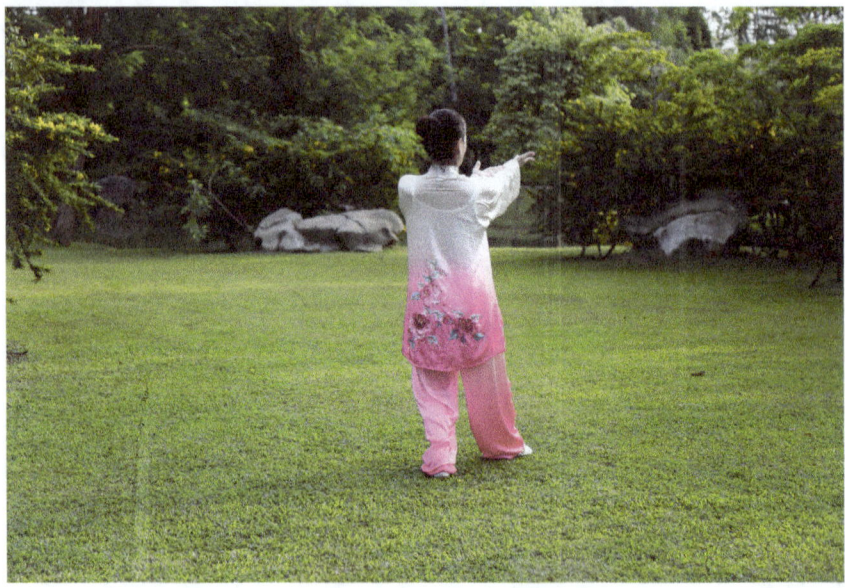

Fig. 6.33.

1. The right foot wades out and the right palm slips out, both toward the northeast direction, palm facing up. Keep the right arm close to straight. At the same time, turn the left palm anti-clockwise until facing up, and then place it on the upper arm (Fig. 6.33).

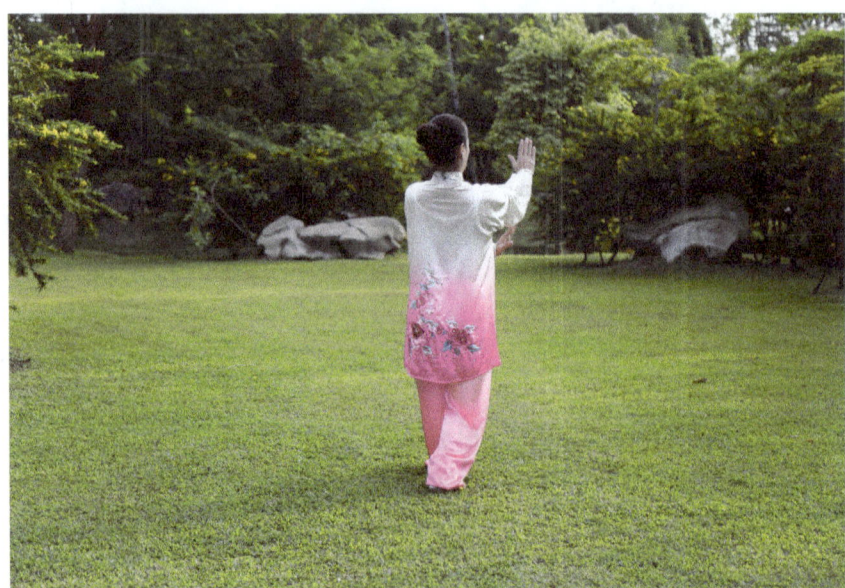

Fig. 6.34.

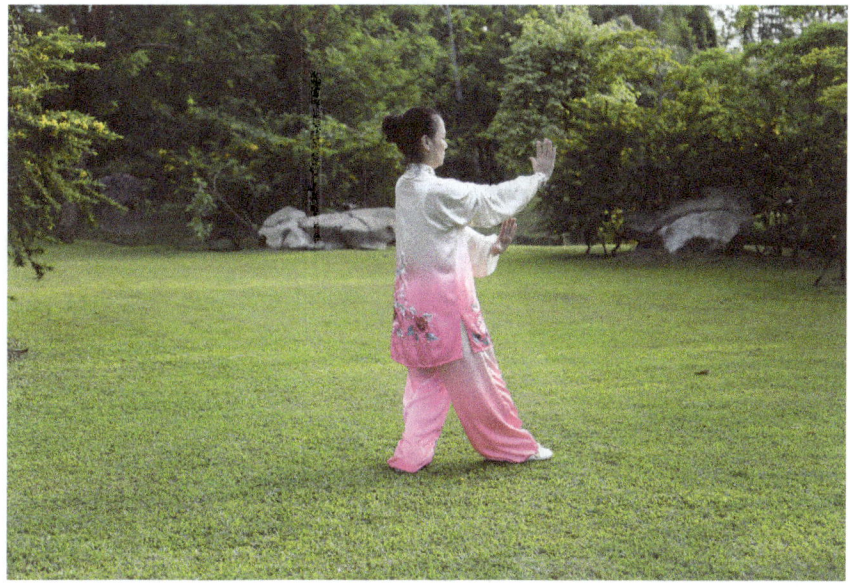

Fig. 6.35.

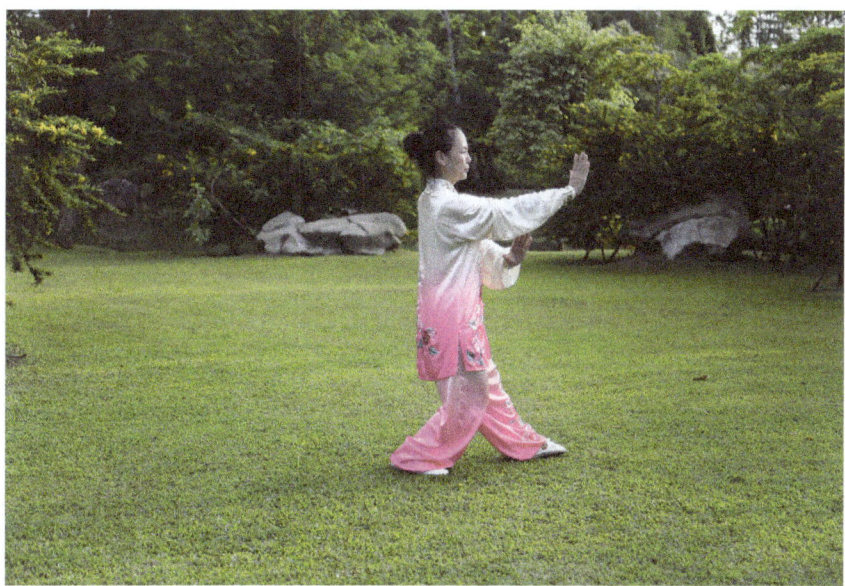

Fig. 6.36.

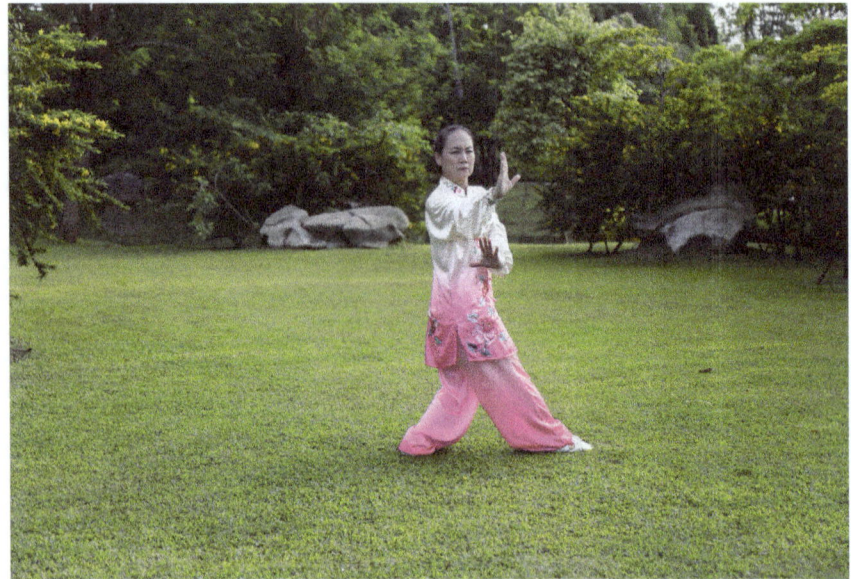

Fig. 6.37.

2. Walk in an arc toward the northeast and north direction with wading steps. At the same time, turn both hands gradually until the palms face out, and push outward while waving rightward. After finishing four steps, stop with the right foot in front and pointing to the east. Both hands should push toward north. The left palm sinks behind the right elbow. Face the direction of the right hand (Figs. 6.34–6.37).

Key Points

Another variation of this form is to finish the arms portion in step 1 without the footwork, and then move the right foot and finish the rightward push of the palms when the right foot touches the ground (just like the hand movements shown in Fig. 6.37). This is then followed by four steps of wading to finish, as Fig. 6.37 illustrates.

11. Inward-latching step with shielding elbow

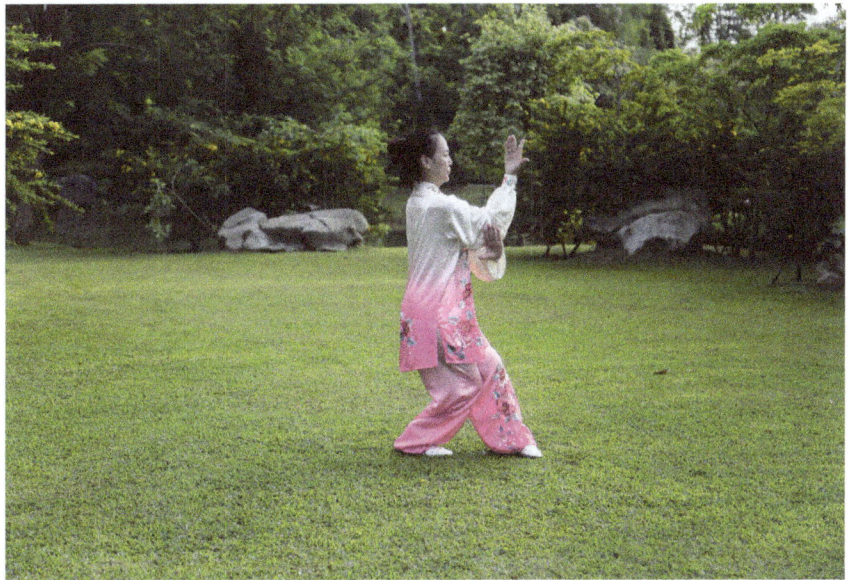

Fig. 6.38.

Move the left foot move forward, just passing the right toe with an inward-latching step. At the same time, the upper body turns left, led by the right shoulder, to form a twist to the left. The right forearm turns anti-clockwise and moves to the left, while the right elbow presses down, with the right upper arm folded until touching the chest. Keep the right forearm in a vertical position and the right palm facing right. The back side of the left palm touches the outside of the right upper arm. Look in direction of the right hand (Fig. 6.38).

Key Points

Maintain the twisted position of the whole body. The arms stay close as if they are to hug together. The right forearm and the right hand need to roll extensively while performing the shielding elbow.

12. Right stealthy tuck-in backward palm

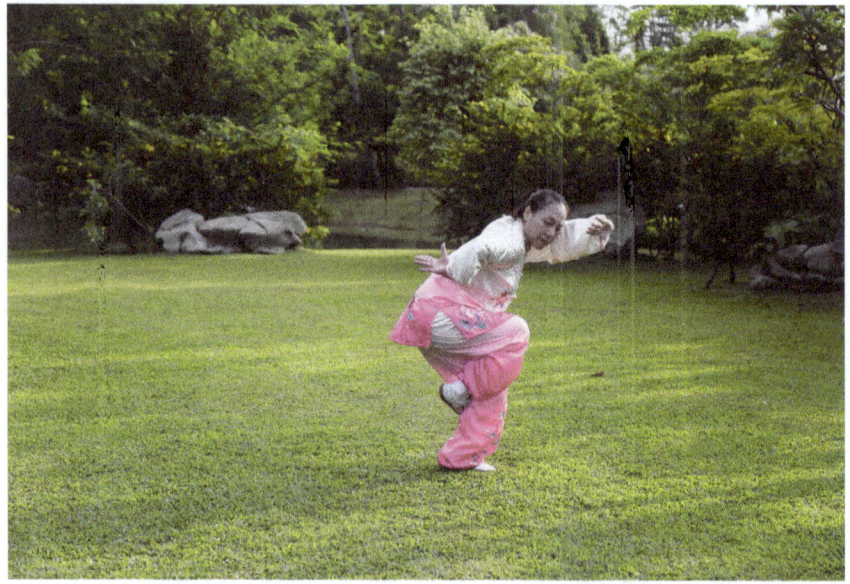

Fig. 6.39.

1. Continue to bend the left leg so as to lower the center of gravity. Lift the right leg with knee folded. The right palm and forearm keep the twisting momentum and slip along the chest, thrusting toward the lower right direction. In the process, the right hand should fold in front of the chest, twisting the wrist in an inward spiral to point the right, keeping the fingers rightward, right palm facing up and tilted at the right rib area. At the same time, the left hand swings naturally toward upper left and stops beside the head, left palm facing left (Fig. 6.39).

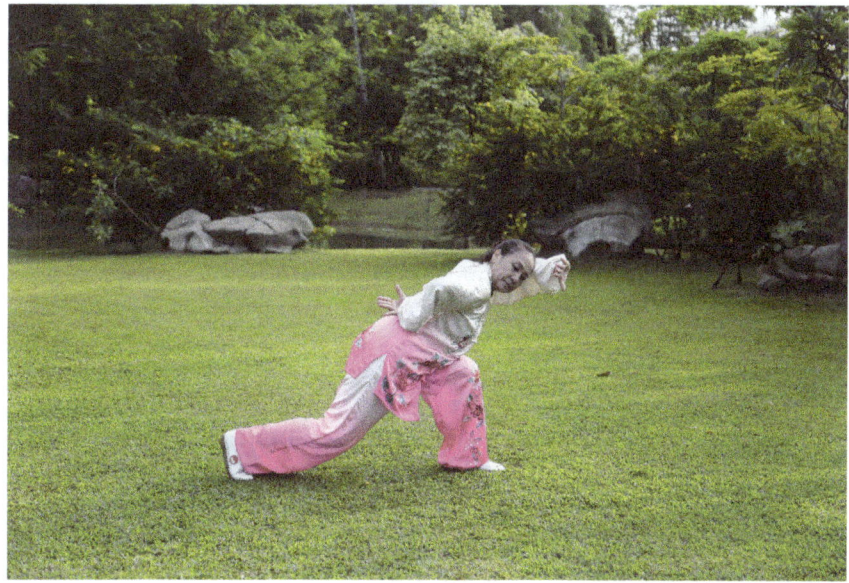

Fig. 6.40.

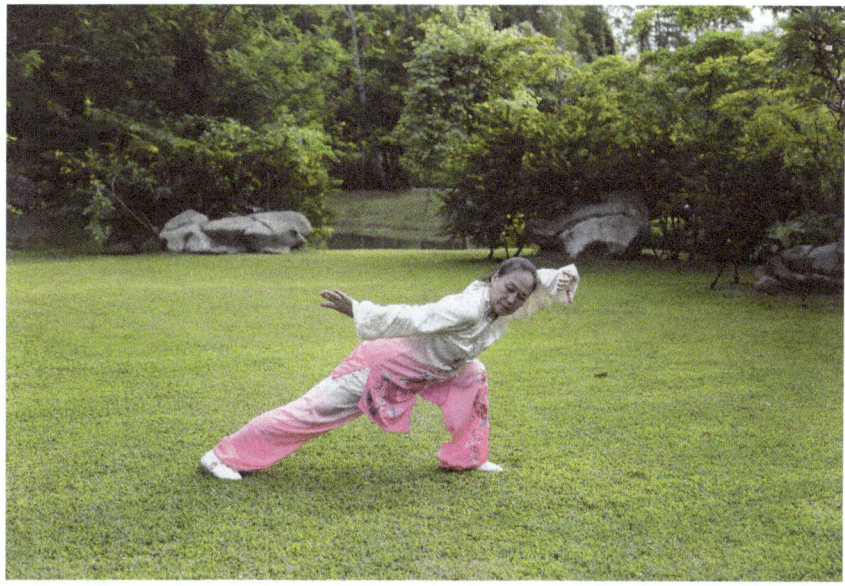

Fig. 6.41.

Next, the right foot strides rightward (west), and at the same time the right palm tucks out rightward, palm facing up (Figs. 6.40–6.41).

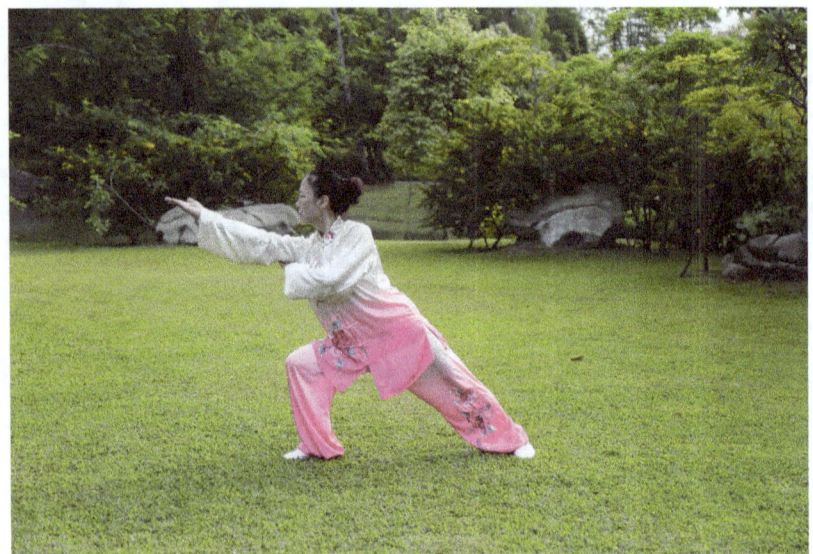

Fig. 6.42.

2. Push off with the left leg to move the center of gravity rightward. Keep the right palm tucking rightward without stopping and move the center of gravity to the right leg, turning the right hand clockwise to face upward. At the same time, the left hand slips toward the right armpit (Fig. 6.42).

13. Forward-step piercing palm

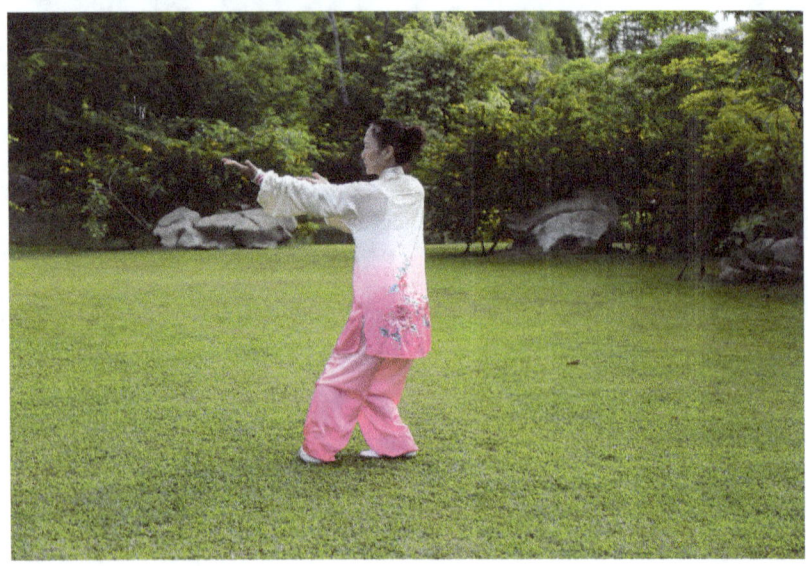

Fig. 6.43.

The left foot quickly steps rightward (west); the foot should latch inward. At the same time, the left palm slips forward from under the right upper arm facing up, at the same height as the shoulders. Simultaneously, the right palm withdraws to the front of the chest facing up. Keep looking in the direction of the left hand (Fig. 6.43).

14. Right-turn cover palm

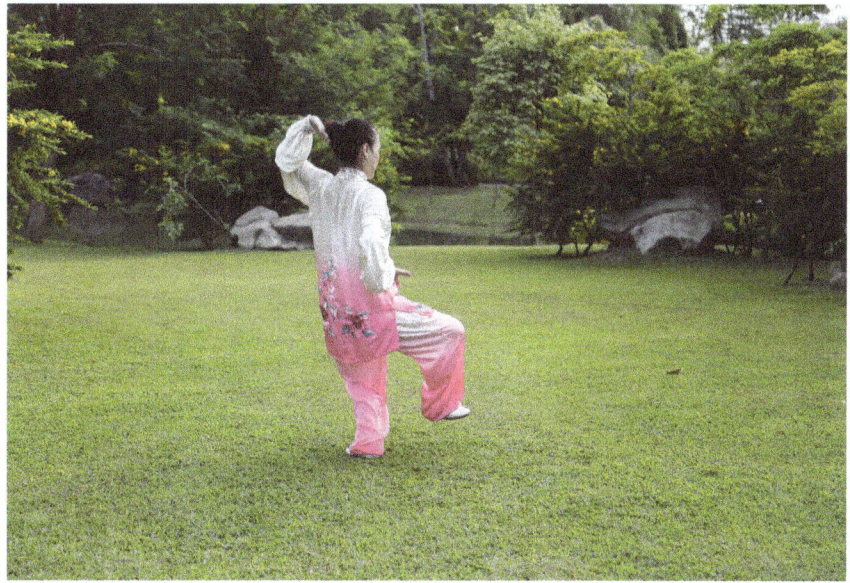

Fig. 6.44.

1. Turn left and lift the right foot with toes pointed to the right side. At the same time, the left arm folds with the left hand stopping behind the head, while the right hand slides down passing the chest and reaches the right waist, palm facing up. The head should turn right (Fig. 6.44).

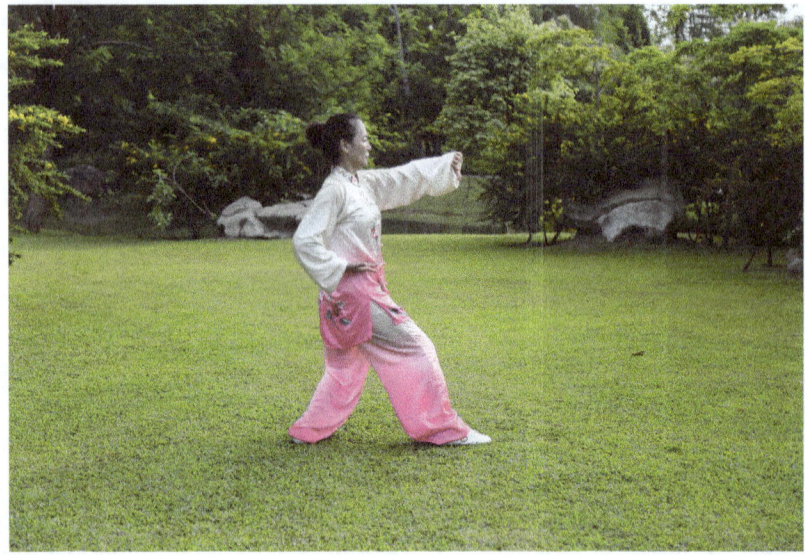

Fig. 6.45.

2. The right foot lands and the left palm covers from above the head and moves forward (east), and then downward, the elbow protruding naturally with the bend of the left arm, with the left palm facing forward (Fig. 6.45).

15. Stride and tuck-in striking palm

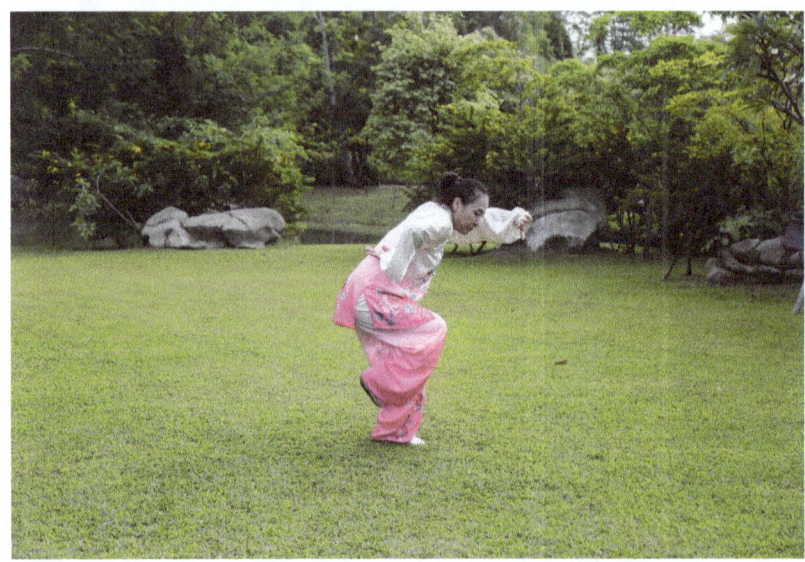

Fig. 6.46.

1. Step forward with the left leg (east), while lifting the right leg. The upper body folds and leans forward. The right palm keeps twisting the wrist in an inward spiral to point to the right, keeping the fingers rightward and the right palm facing up (Fig. 6.46).

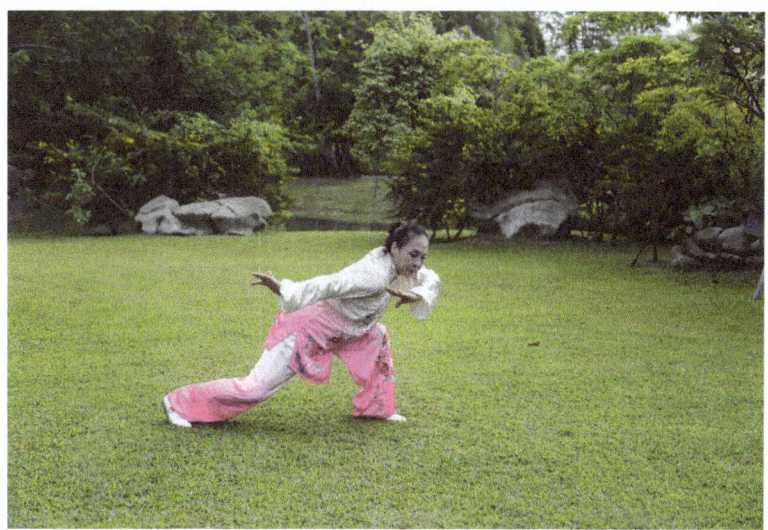

Fig. 6.47.

2. Next, the right foot strides toward the west, with the right palm tucking out toward the west, along the right waist and right side of the back, arm finishing straight and palm facing up (Fig. 6.47).

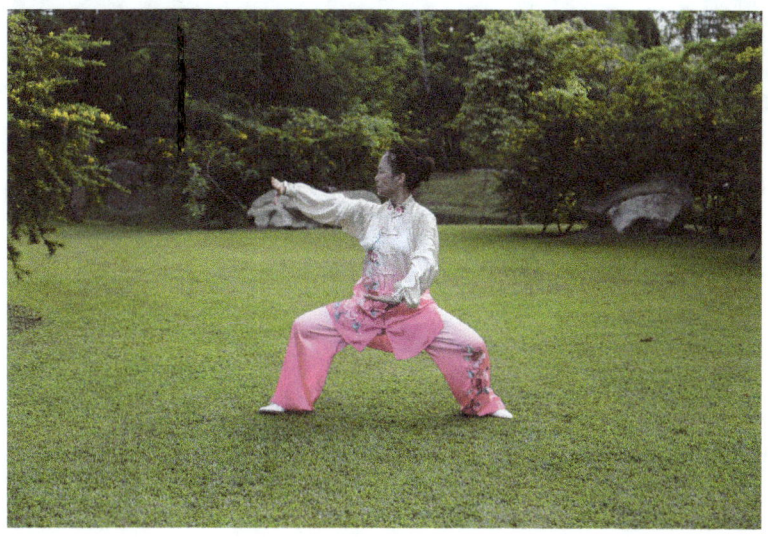

Fig. 6.48.

Shift the center of the body weight in between the two feet, and thrust the right wrist toward the right, with the right palm facing right. The right heel is the major attacking point. The right arm is leveled with the right shoulder. The left hand should push down in an arc and stop in front of the belly button. Look to the right (Fig. 6.48).

Key Points

1. The tuck-in, which comes before the strike, should be flexible, but the strike needs to be very powerful.
2. At the beginning of training, the focus should be on the right path of the movement and handwork, not the power. The power will be released gradually when the form is polished.

16. Turn with whirling arms

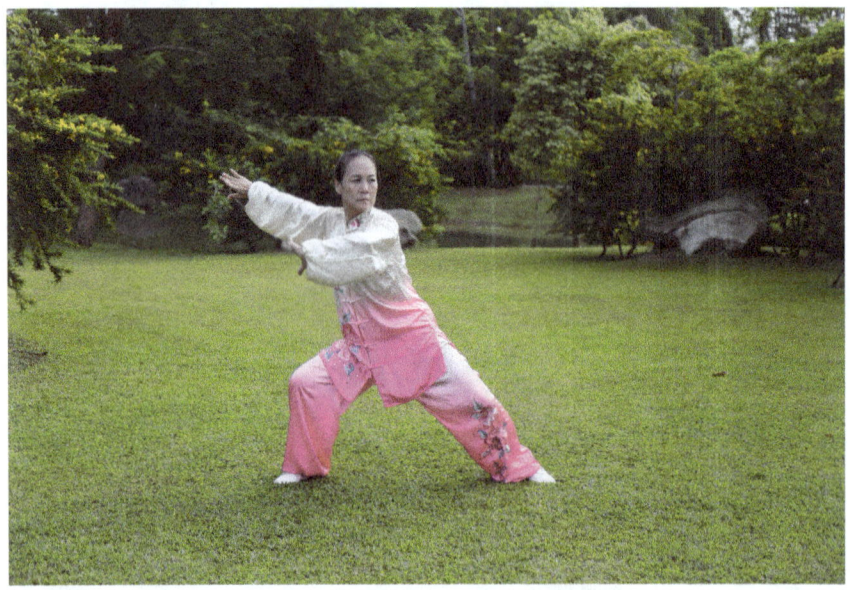

Fig. 6.49.

1. The body shifts slightly rightward while turning right. The arms swing to the right with the body, and the head turns to the left (Fig. 6.49).

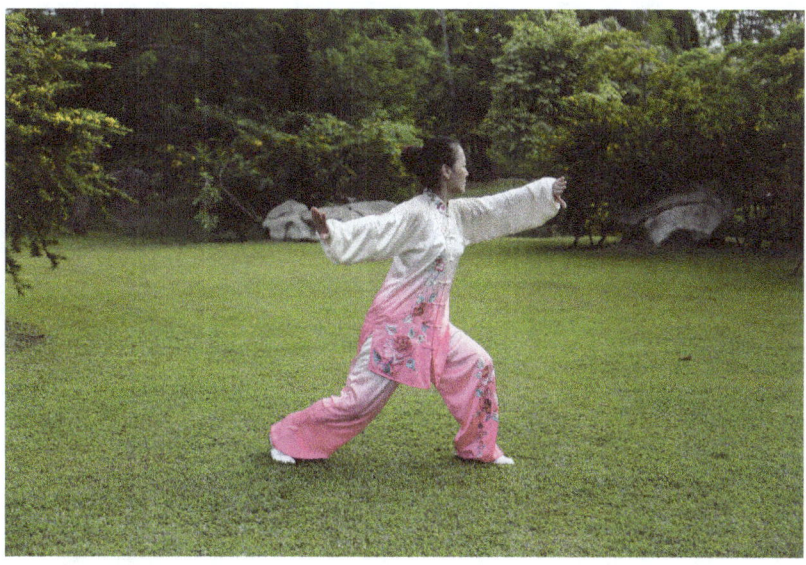

Fig. 6.50.

2. Next, quickly turn the body left. The center of gravity shifts to the left while the left arm waves to the left with the spinning of the body. Both hands should be fisted, and the back of the fists should face back behind the body (Fig. 6.50).

17. Back-hand thump

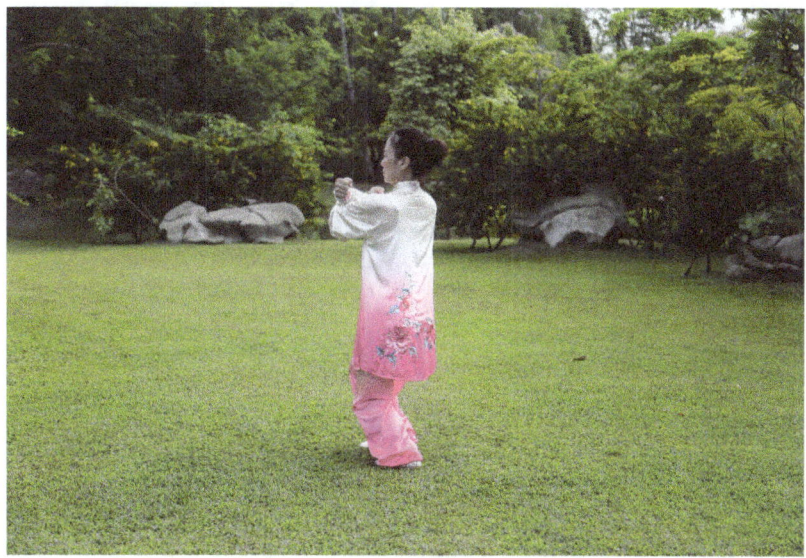

Fig. 6.51.

1. Keep turning left without stopping, and move the right foot forward quickly to get close to the left foot. At the same time, fold the arms into a hug in front of the body, palms facing behind the body in fists (Fig. 6.51).

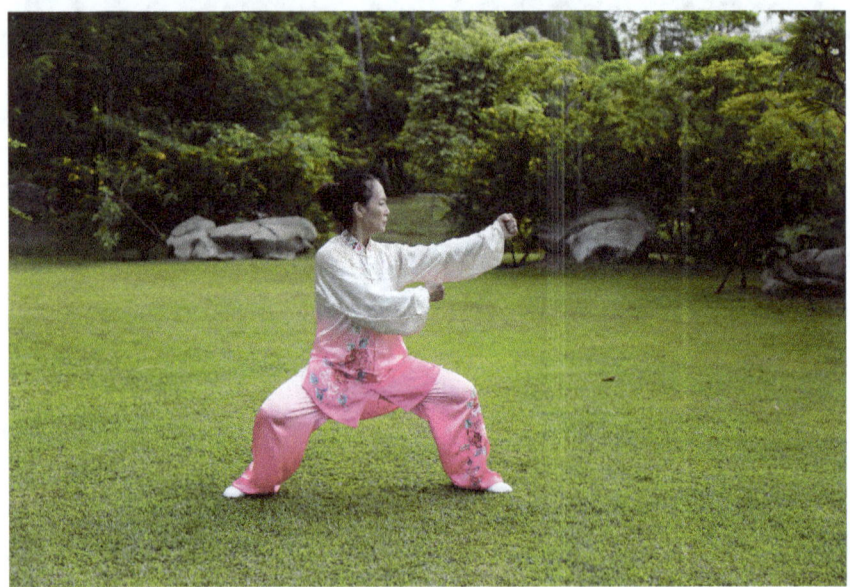

Fig. 6.52.

2. Keep turning left without stopping, and stride backward quickly with the right foot to form a horse stance with the chest facing south. While the left foot is landing, the left arm flexes and swings quickly to the left (Fig. 6.52).

Key Points

1. Forms 16 and 17 should be completed continuously without any stops, with high speed and great power.
2. Sink into the horse stance immediately with the landing of the left foot. However, for beginners, you may land both feet together to find better balancing, in this case, there is a sound when the feet land.

18. Cloud hand right tuck-in palm

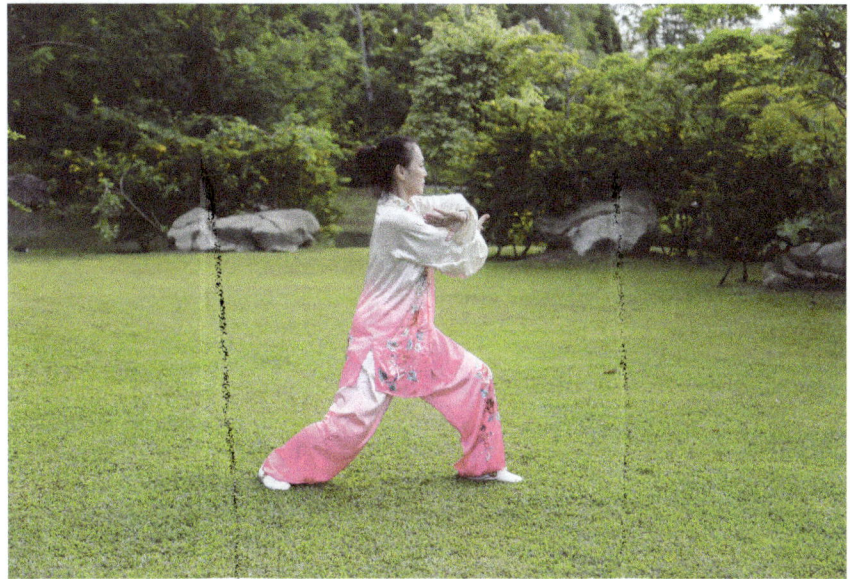

Fig. 6.53.

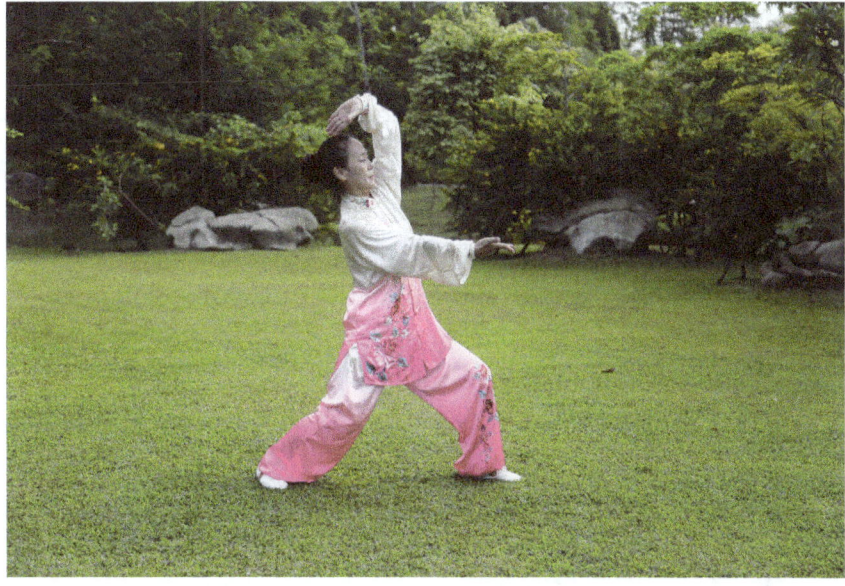

Fig. 6.54.

1. Wave both hands above the head to perform a wide right cloud hand: the left hand waves toward the upper right, and then backward in a circle; at the same time, the right hand circles toward the right side from below the left arm (Figs. 6.53–6.54).

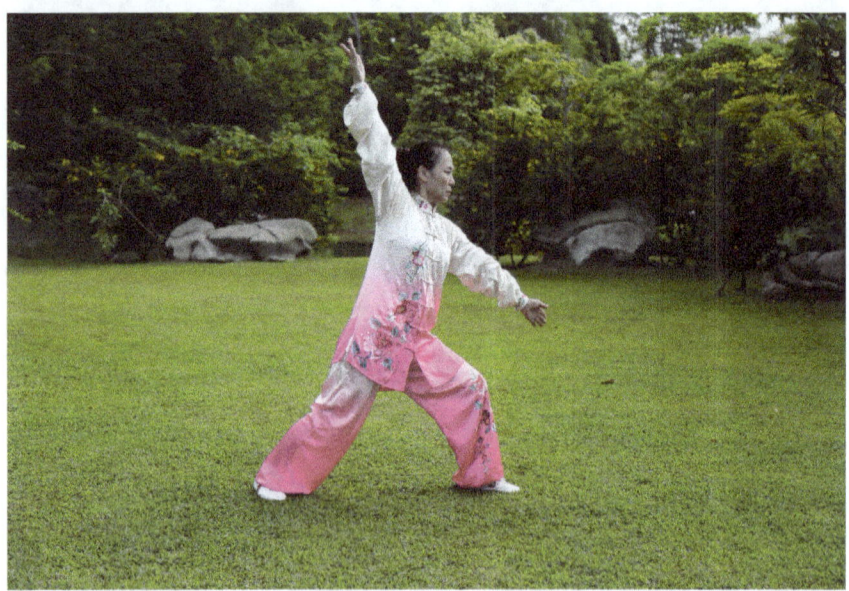

Fig. 6.55.

The left hand continues to circle toward the left and front. At the same time, the right hand continues to wave backward, and then upward in an arc (Fig. 6.55).

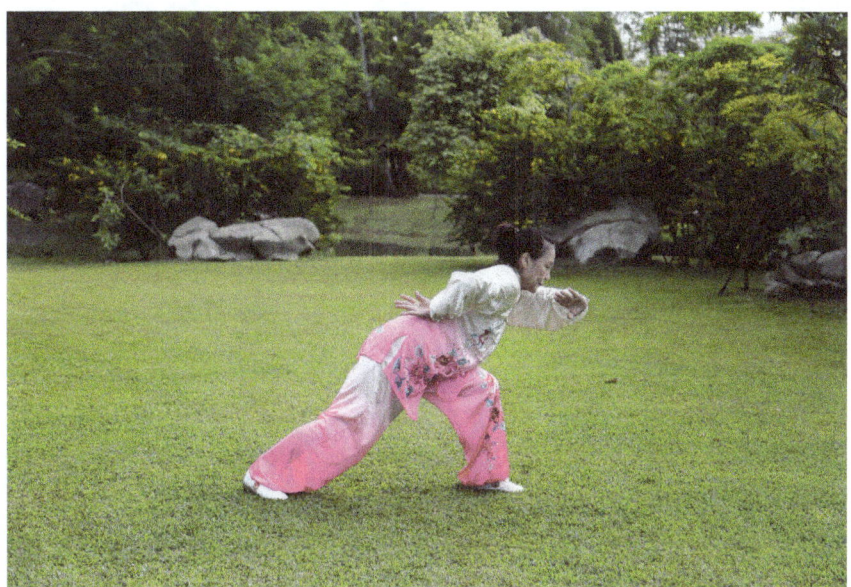

Fig. 6.56.

2. Without stopping, the right arm folds with the wrist twisting in an inward spiral to have the right palm tucked out backward, fingers pointed backward and thrust backward along the right waist, palm facing up (Fig. 6.56).

Key Points

The form should be performed at one go with a wide range.

19. Turning cloud palm

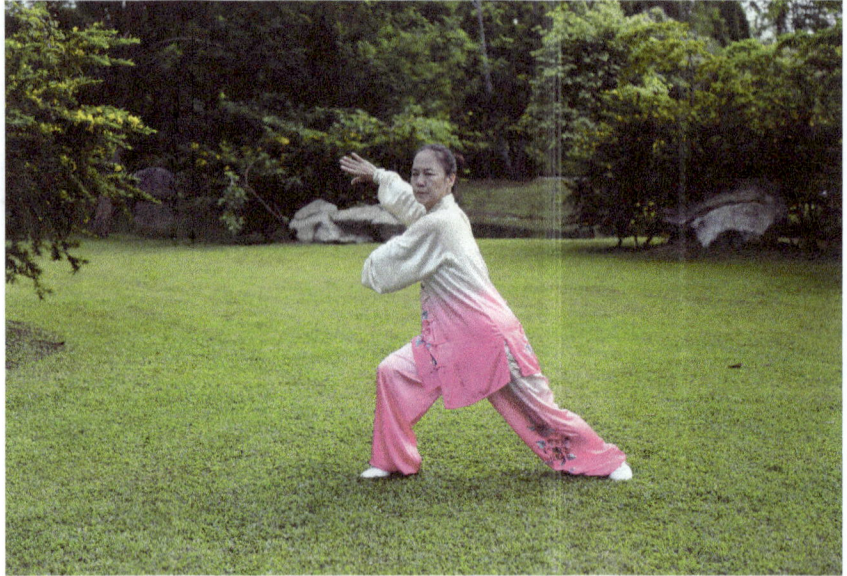

Fig. 6.57.

1. The center of gravity of the body moves to the right, and the right hand extends further rightward. At the same time, the left hand swings rightward to reach the right rib area (Fig. 6.57).

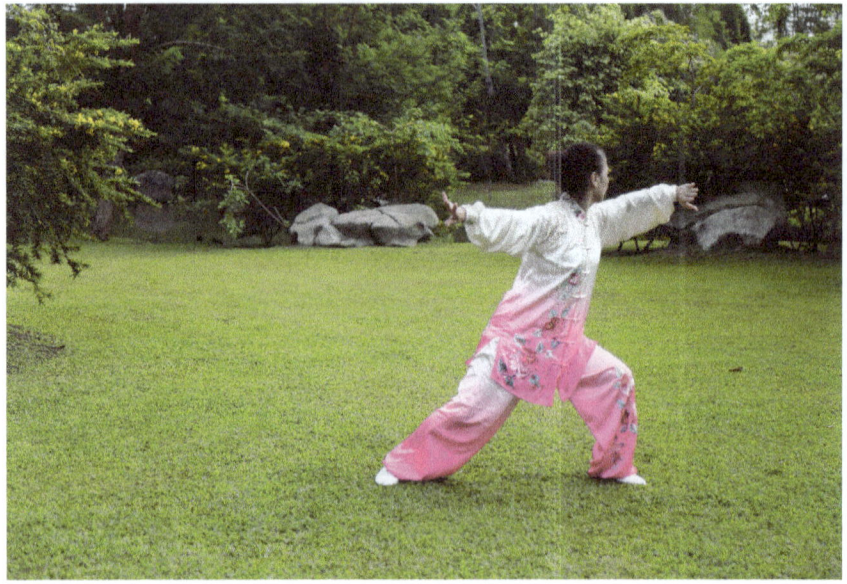

Fig. 6.58.

2. The center of gravity of the body moves to the left, which pulls the left hand to wave forward and then leftward in a circle (Fig. 6.58).

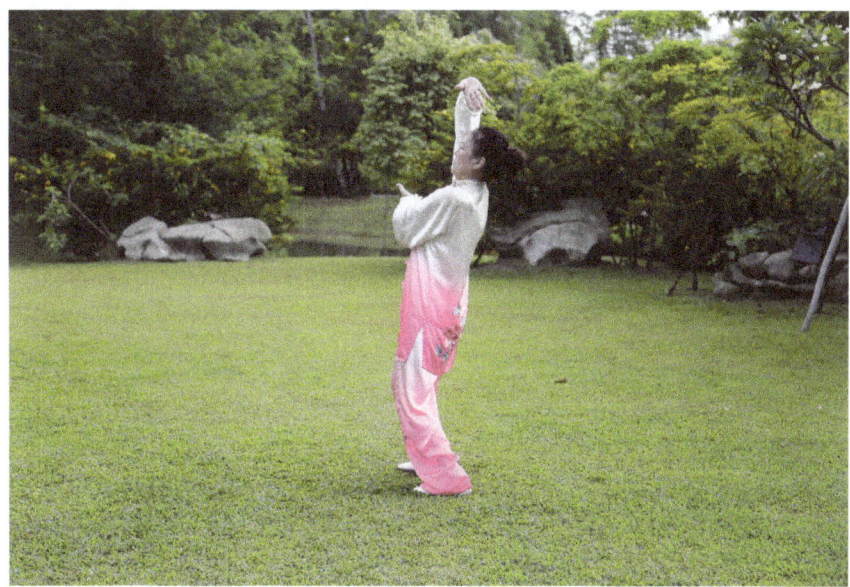

Fig. 6.59.

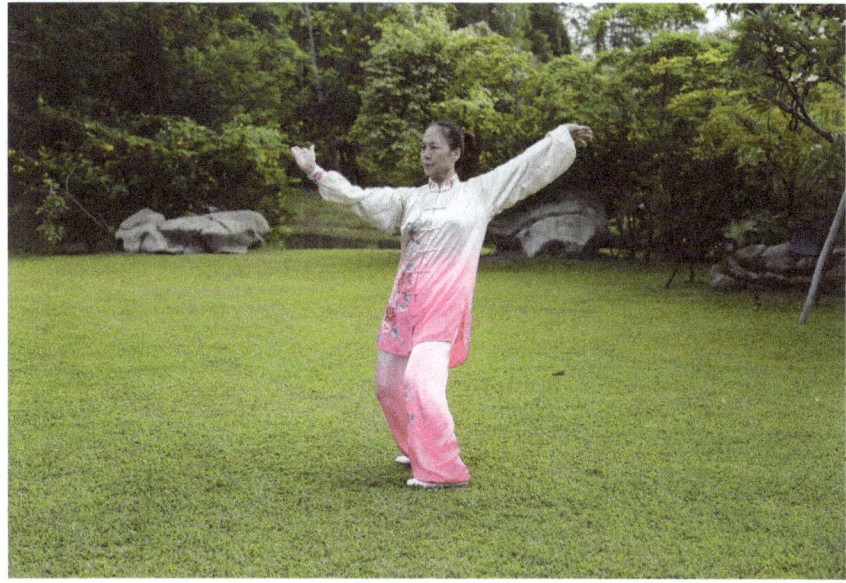

Fig. 6.60.

3. The left foot points outward while the right foot moves quickly forward and then toward the left backside (which is going east and then north and then west) to perform an inward-latching step in a circle. At the same time, tilt the head back slightly and wave both hands above the head to quickly perform a wide left cloud hand, which is to wave the right hand toward the left for two rounds in a circle. At the same time, the left arm bends to circle toward the left side for one round from below the right arm (Figs. 6.59 and 6.60).

20. Squat hugging palm

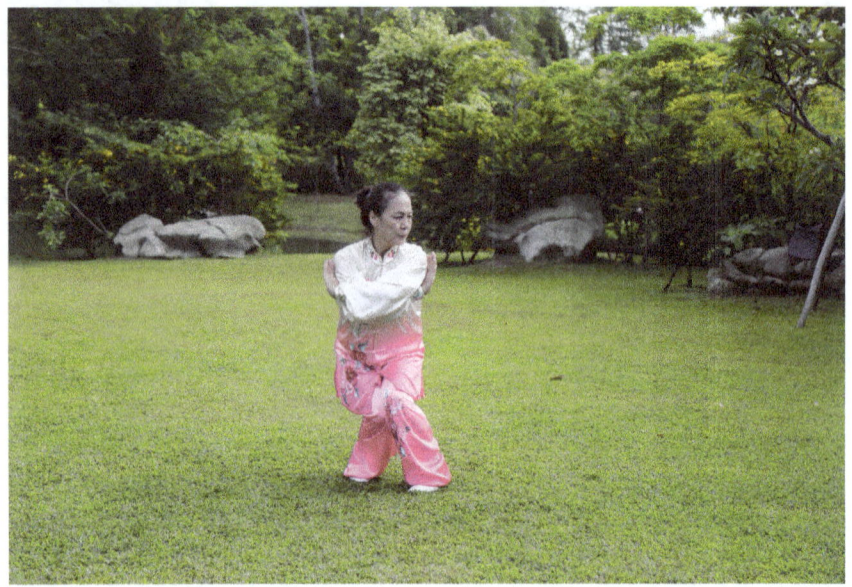

Fig. 6.61.

Squat down quickly, hugging with both arms at once (Fig. 6.61).

21. Piercing palm with left knee lifted

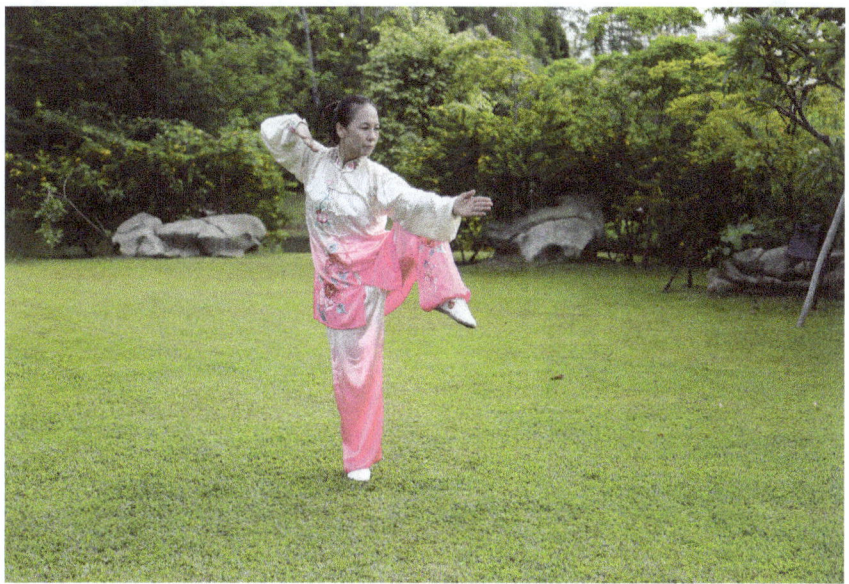

Fig. 6.62.

Push off forcefully with the right leg and stand up quickly with the left knee lifted. At the same time, the left palm pierces toward the lower left quickly and forcefully, keeping the wrist straight and fingers closed. The right palm pulls back in front of the right shoulder, palm facing down. Maintain this stance for a while and gaze toward the left hand (Fig. 6.62).

Key Points

The two forms above should be completed with wide range, great speed, and great power.

22. Forward right thrust palm

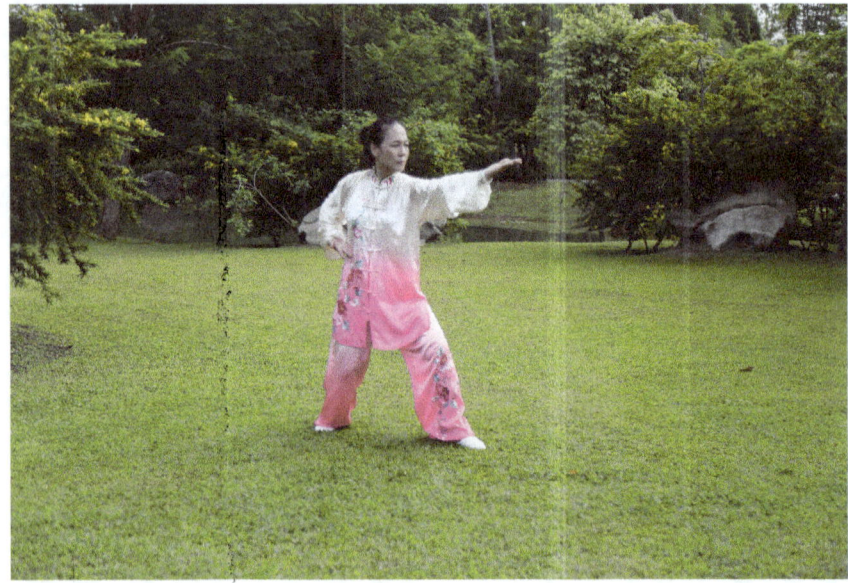

Fig. 6.63.

1. The left foot lands naturally and the right hand comes down to the side of the right rib, palms facing up (Fig. 6.63).

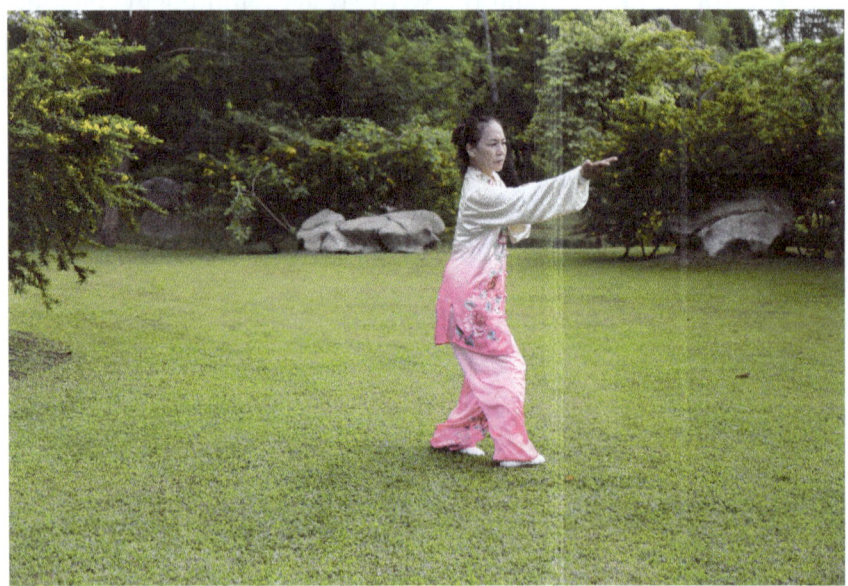

Fig. 6.64.

2. Next, the right foot steps forward to perform an inward-latching step. At the same time, the right palm thrusts forward, palm facing up. The left hand pulls back from below the right arm to the right chest. Gaze toward the right palm (Fig. 6.64).

23. Turn to thrust palm left and right

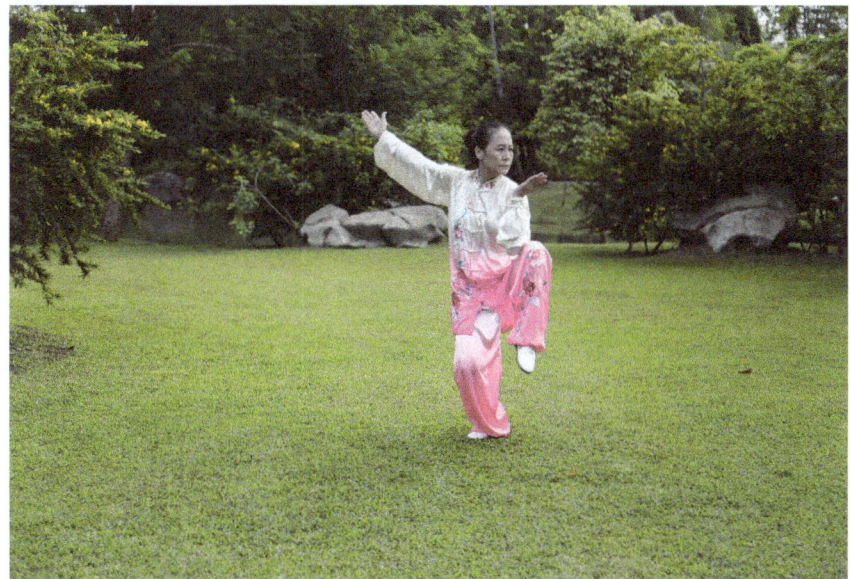

Fig. 6.65.

1. Without stopping, turn left with the left foot lifted, chest facing south while looking at the east. At the same time, the left palm moves to the front of the left shoulder to under the chin, palm facing up, left fingers pointing to the east. The right arm extends to the west with the turning of the body (Fig. 6.65).

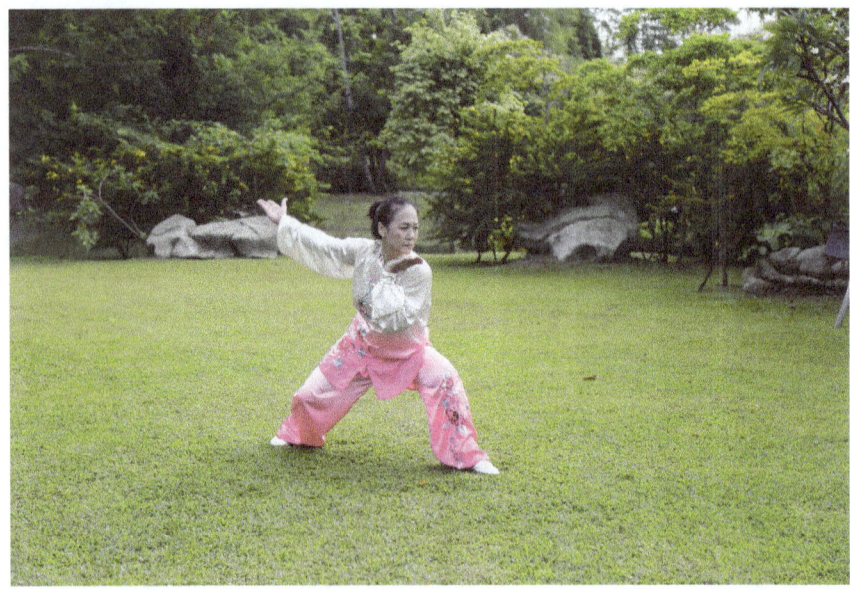

Fig. 6.66.

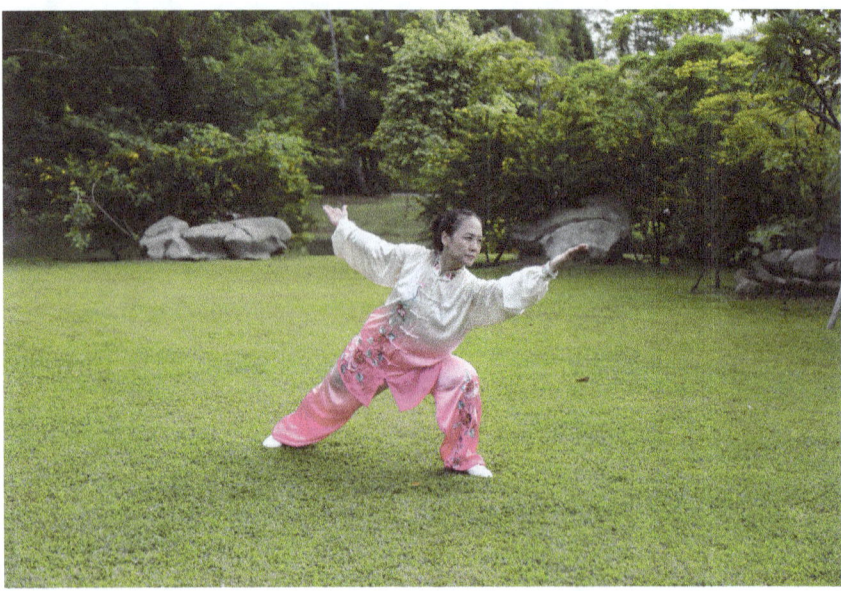

Fig. 6.67.

2. The left foot lands toward the east or a little southeast, and the left palm thrusts toward the left, keeping the two arms nearly in one line, palms facing up. The upper body leans toward the east as much as possible. Gaze toward the left palm (Figs. 6.66 and 6.67).

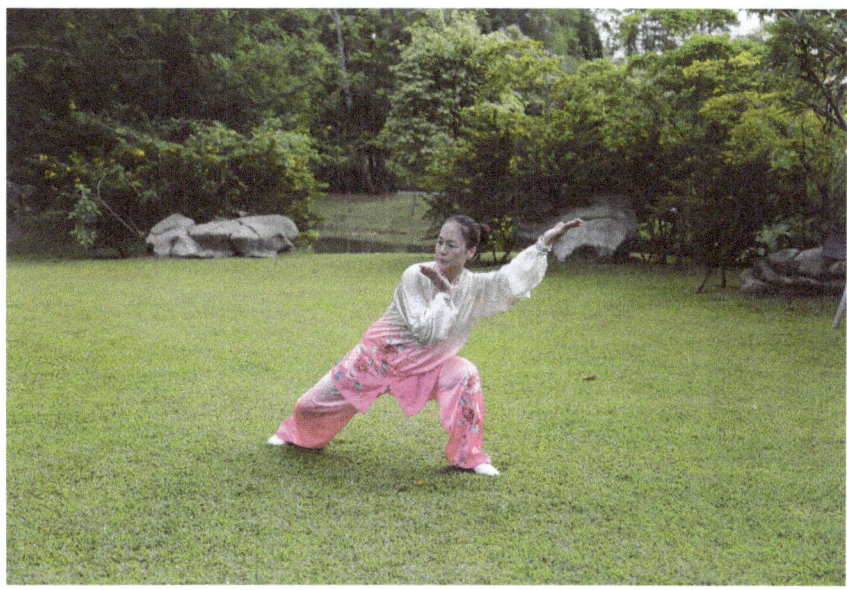

Fig. 6.68.

3. The fingers point to the right side, and the head turns to the right (Fig. 6.68).

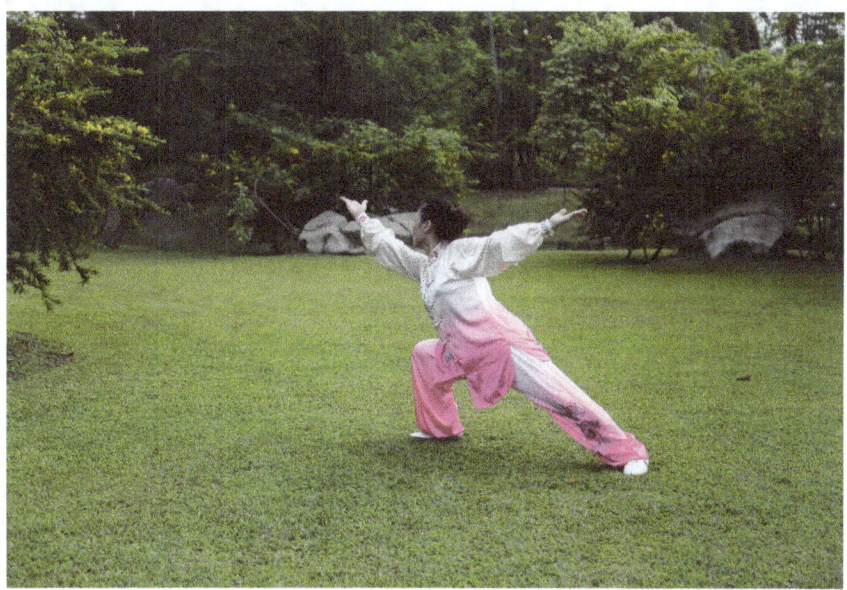

Fig. 6.69.

Push off forcefully with the left leg and move the body to the right. At the same time, the right palm thrusts toward the right, palms facing up. The upper body leans toward the right as much as possible. Gaze toward the right palm (Fig. 6.69).

Key Points

1. The shifting of the center of gravity between the left and right should be fast with a wide range.
2. The palms always thrust from under the chin without using too much force. The thrust of the palms should be flexible and yet strongly connected with the body movement without any pause.
3. This form should be practiced multiple times to achieve perfection.

24. Backward-leaning plane turning palm

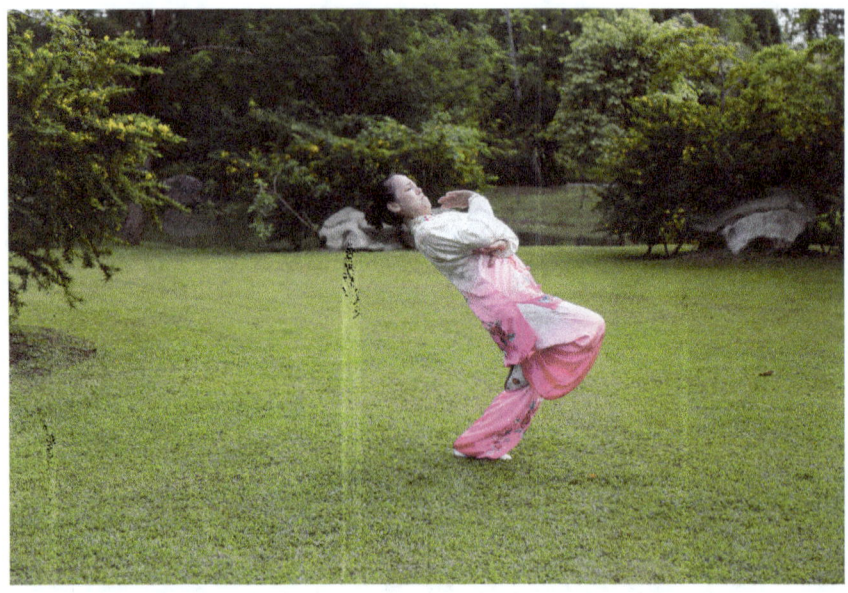

Fig. 6.70.

1. Push off with the right leg and move the body weight to the left leg, and turn left. The right foot starts to move forward (east or a little southeast). In the process, the right instep touches the left knee from behind, leaning the upper body backward. At the same time, the right palm turns in a horizontal plane clockwise, which is from back to the

front (and from the right to the left). Fold the elbow to keep the right palm in a clockwise plane turning movement, palms facing up. At the same time, the left arm bends with the left palm touching the lower part of the right upper arm. Keep the left palm facing down while gazing forward (Fig. 6.70).

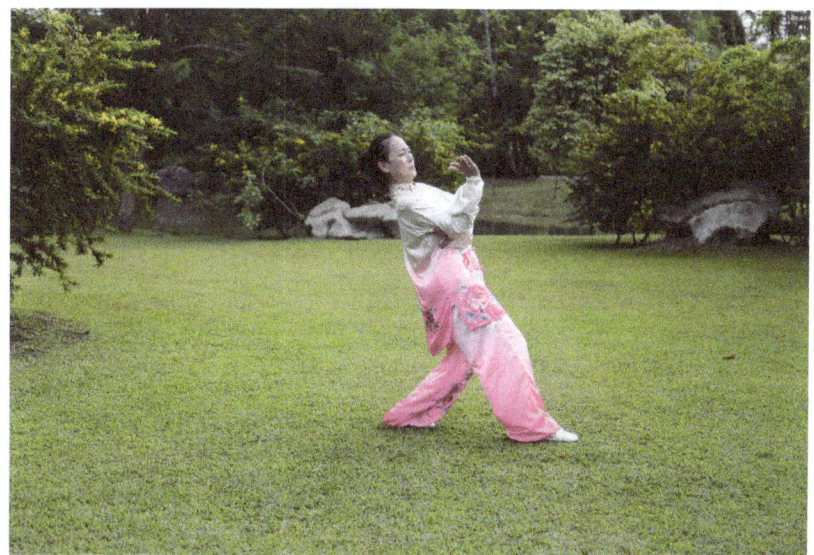

Fig. 6.71.

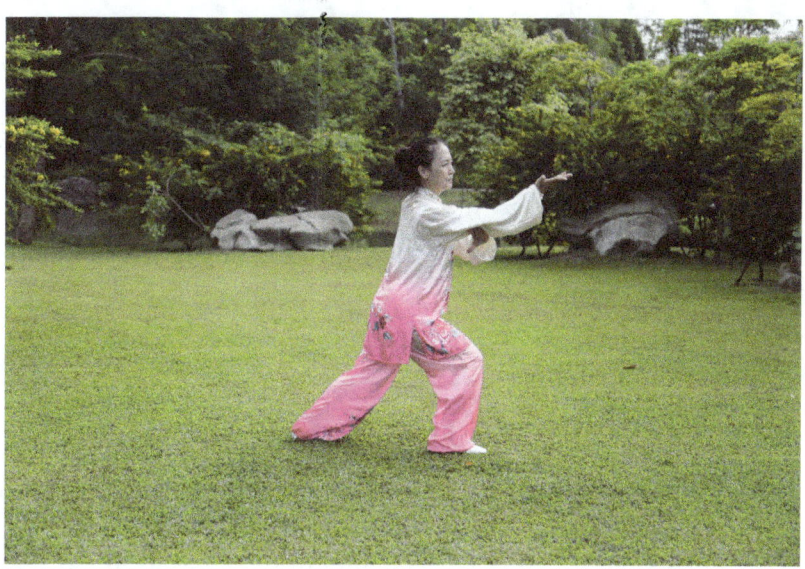

Fig. 6.72.

2. The right foot lands with the body weight moving forward, and at the same time, the right hand continues the circular waving to the right and then to the front and end up forming a leftward chopping palm in front of the body. The right arm bends slightly, palm facing up. The power-releasing point is at the side of the right little finger (Figs. 6.71 and 6.72).

Key Points

1. The forward waving of the right arm should be wide, and the arm should circle around in front of the body at neck height. While circling, the right hand flips naturally, withdrawing to be close to the body, turning in a horizontal plane and chopping to the left horizontally.
2. Do not practice this form too fast. The form should have power with flexibility, and showcase a type of inner power and unity of the whole body strength.

25. Withdraw step tuck-in palm

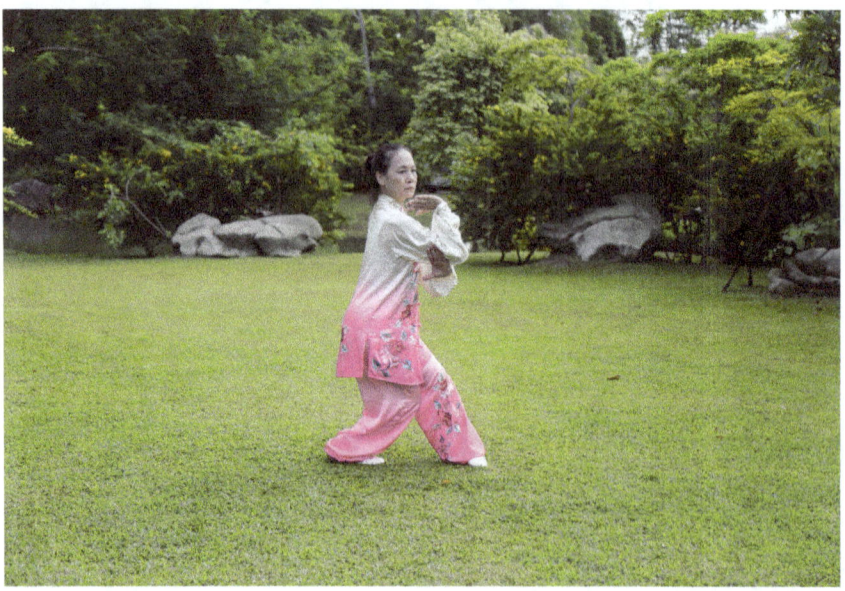

Fig. 6.73.

1. The left foot moves forward to form an inward-latching step. At the same time, the right arm folds quickly. Withdraw the right palm in front of the right shoulder, palm facing up, fingers pointing to the back side, while the left palm stays under the upper right arm (Fig. 6.73).

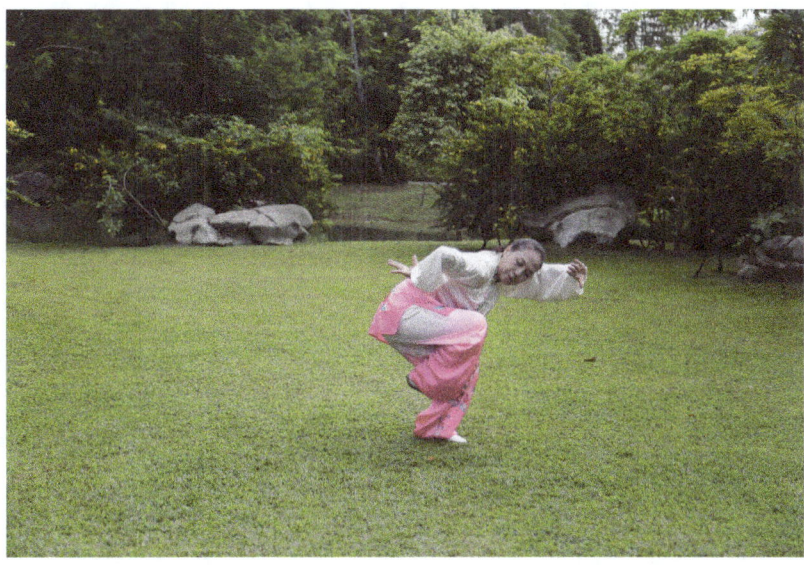

Fig. 6.74.

2. The right leg lifts up, while the upper body folds and leans forward. At the same time, the right palm keeps twisting the wrist in an inward spiral to point to the right, keeping the fingers rightward, right palm facing up and tilted at the right rib area, while preparing to thrust backward. At the same time, the left hand swings naturally forward, and the head turns right (Fig. 6.74).

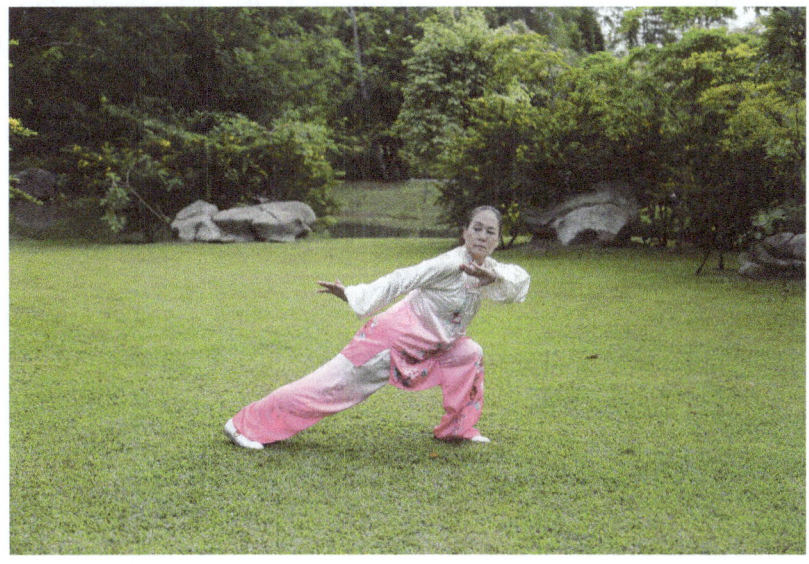

Fig. 6.75.

Next, the right foot strides backward, the right palm tucks out backward, the right arm finishes straight, while the left palm starts to fold back to the front of the chest (Fig. 6.75).

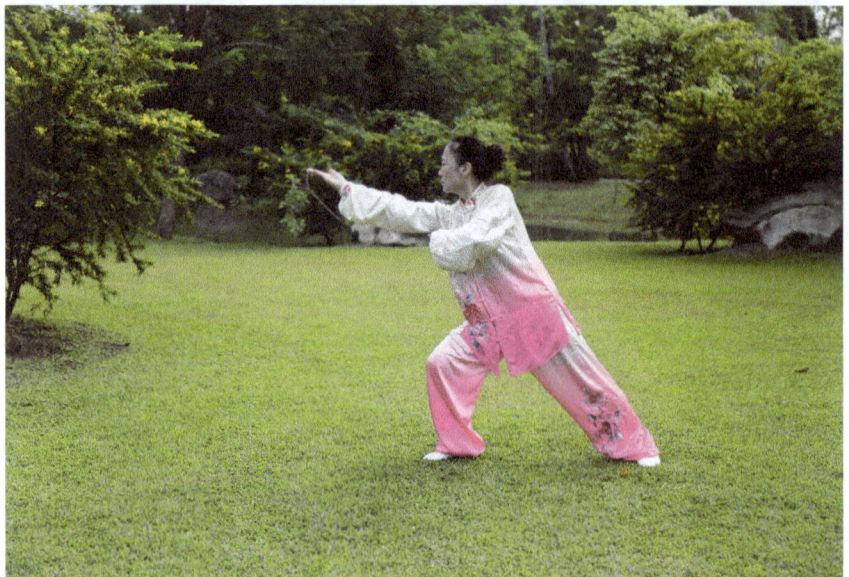

Fig. 6.76.

3. Push off with the left leg to move the center of gravity rightward and turn right. Keep thrusting the right palm toward the west while spinning clockwise. The left hand slips below the right upper arm. Gaze toward the right hand (Fig. 6.76).

Key Points

1. While practicing, the first step of this form should be performed seamlessly with the previous form. The whole body should then suddenly shake in a swift and relaxed manner to complete the transition between the forms until the tuck-in palm finishes. This demands a well-trained body extremely good at relaxing. Chinese martial artists often describe Bagua Palm as a wavy stance or dragon-like motion, which more or less describes the style of Bagua Palm. To perform in a true Bagua Palm manner, the ability to relax the whole body is a must.

2. All inner-style martial arts are built on the ability to relax thoroughly, to be relaxed but not soft, to be flexible with strength weaved in so as to reach excellent body coordination. In fact, the external style of Chinese martial arts also demands the ability to relax. Only when relaxed can the strength be built, the release of the force made possible, and application in self-defense and fighting realized. Also, Chinese martial art is not only for self-defense but also for health improvement. The extent of relaxation also decides the effectiveness in health improvement. The relaxed shaking of the body can improve the running of the real *Qi* inside the body and improve health through enhanced circulation.

26. Forward-step piercing palm

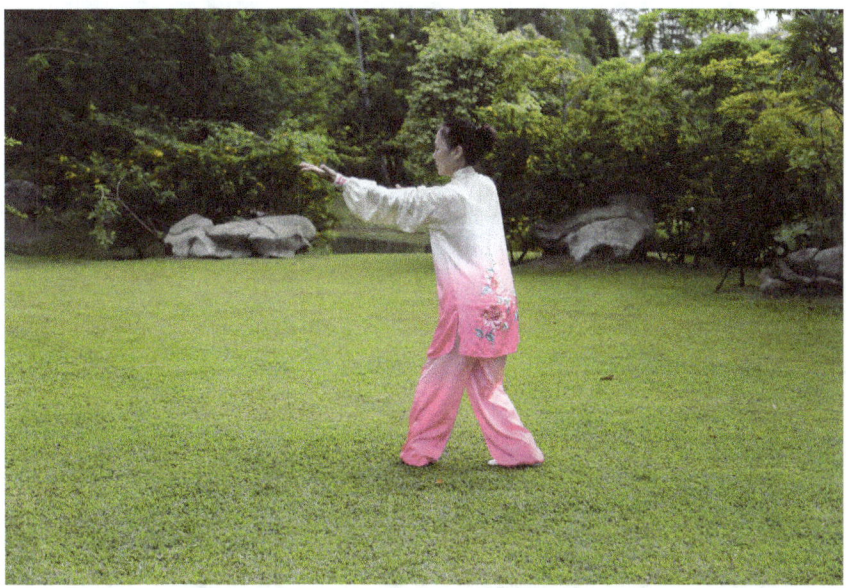

Fig. 6.77.

The left foot moves forward (west) to perform an inward-latching step. The body starts to turn right, and at the same time the left palm pierces from under the right upper arm and along the right arm, palm facing up. The right palm folds back to the left chest, palm facing up. Look toward the left palm (Fig. 6.77).

27. Turn for wiping palm

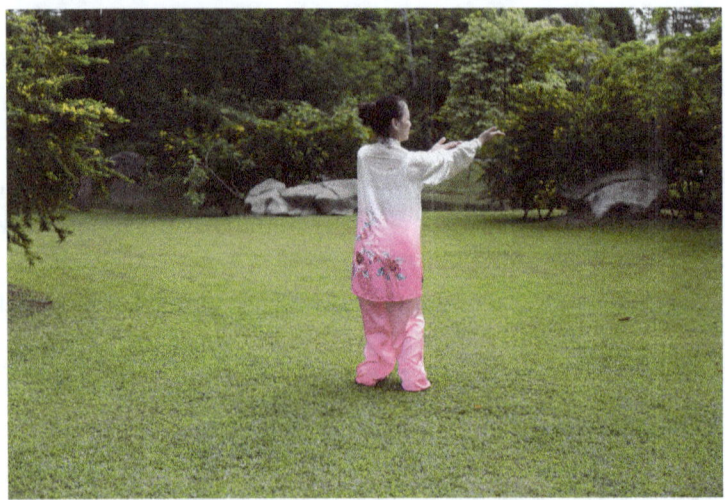

Fig. 6.78.

1. Without stopping, turn right with the left palm waving to the right in an arc. At the same time, the right palm pierces from under the left upper arm and along the left arm. The right arm straightens and waves to the right in a horizontal arc. The left arm folds gradually in the process and withdraws along and above the right upper arm, both palms facing up. Gaze toward the right palm (Fig. 6.78).

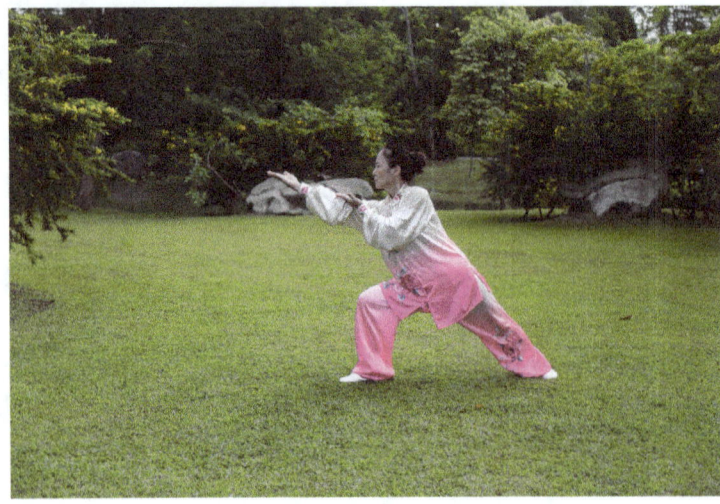

Fig. 6.79.

2. The body continues to turn right. The right foot strides backward (west) and the center of gravity moves to the right leg. The left leg goes straight naturally to form a right bow stance. At the same time, the right arm keeps waving to the right in a horizontal arc and stops eastward. The left palm folds gradually in the process and withdraws to be close to the right upper arm. Gaze toward the right palm (Fig. 6.79).

Key Points

This form needs to be performed with accuracy but not necessarily with much power releasing. It should be connected with the next form.

28. Hugging palms to roll

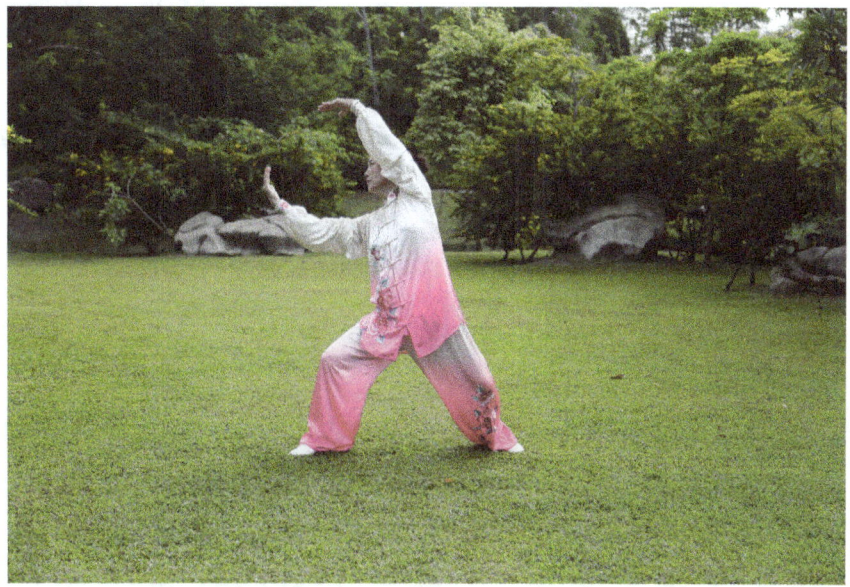

Fig. 6.80.

1. The body weight moves leftward while turning to the left. Both arms extend straight upward and then wave toward the left in an arc (Fig. 6.80).

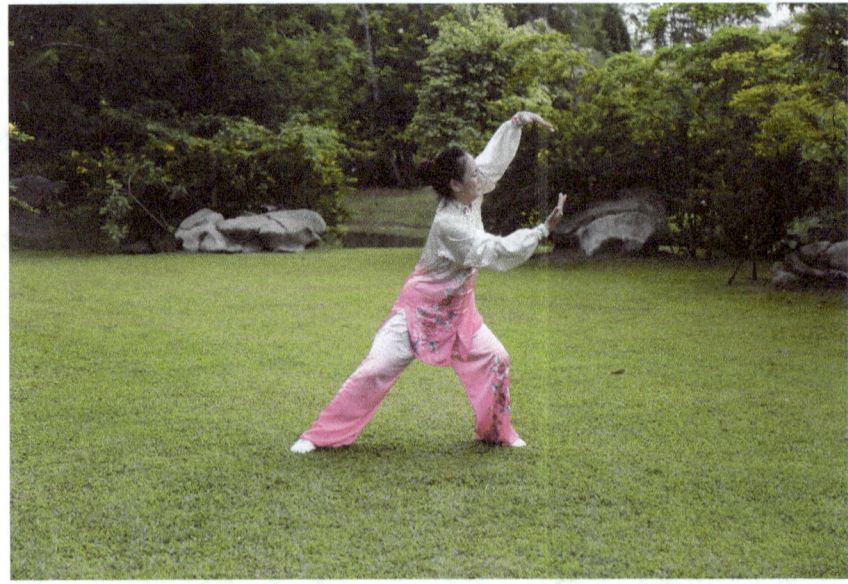

Fig. 6.81.

While the upper body turns to the left, the arms curve to form a hugging posture at the left side of the body with the left palm above the head, the fingers of two hands tilting and pointing to each other. Look toward the upper left side (Fig. 6.81).

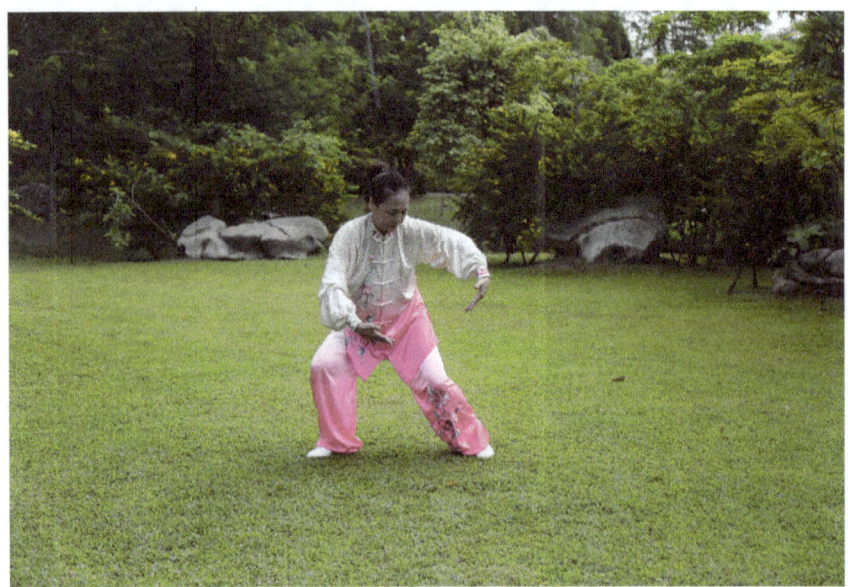

Fig. 6.82.

2. The body weight moves rightward while turning to the right, and both legs bend. At the same time, both arms maintain the hugging posture and then wave down and toward the right in an arc. Look at the space in between the hands (Fig. 6.82).

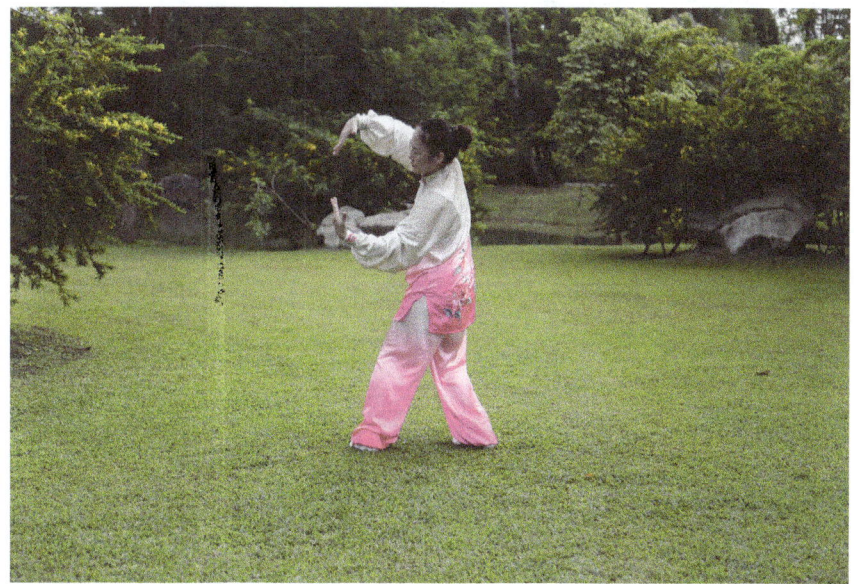

Fig. 6.83.

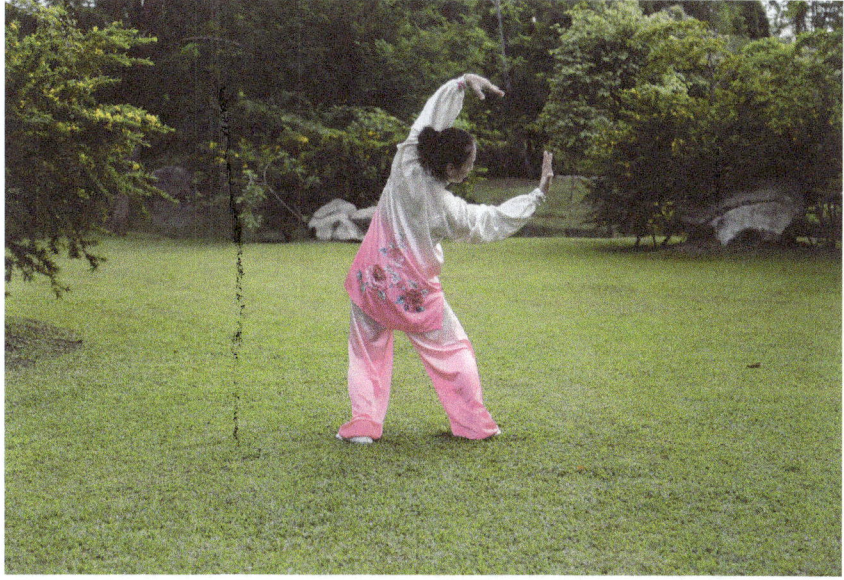

Fig. 6.84.

The left foot steps right (west) and the upper body keeps rolling toward the right. The hip moves forward and the upper body naturally leans back. At the same time, the two arms in their hugging posture keep rotating to the right, upward, and toward the east in an arc until the right upper side is tilted to the east (Figs. 6.83 and 6.84).

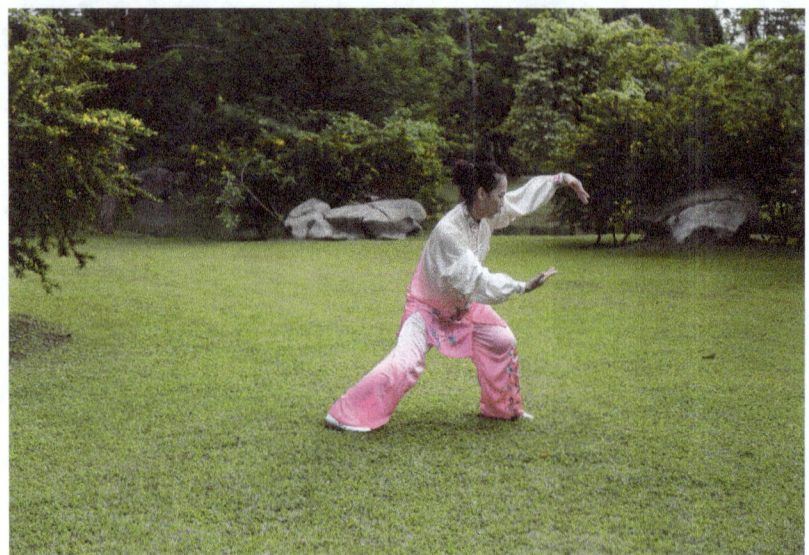

Fig. 6.85.

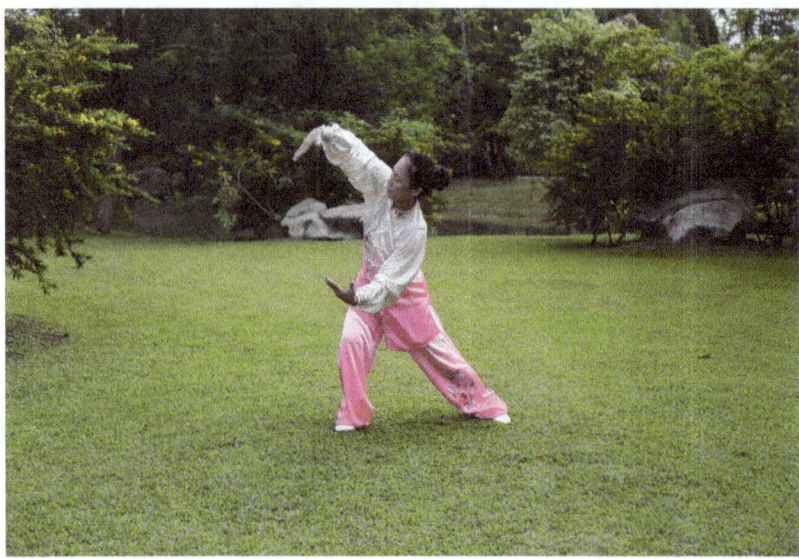

Fig. 6.86.

3. The right foot steps backward (west), the upper body continues to rotate toward the right, the two arms in a hugging posture. Keep rolling downward and then to the right in an arc (Figs. 6.85 and 6.86).

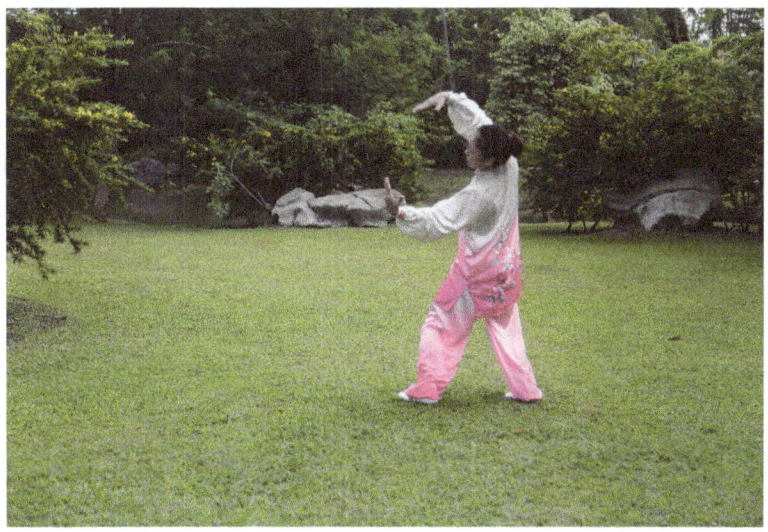

Fig. 6.87.

4. The left foot steps forward to the right and the upper body continues to rotate toward the right. With the two arms in a hugging posture, keep rotating upward in an arc (Fig. 6.87).

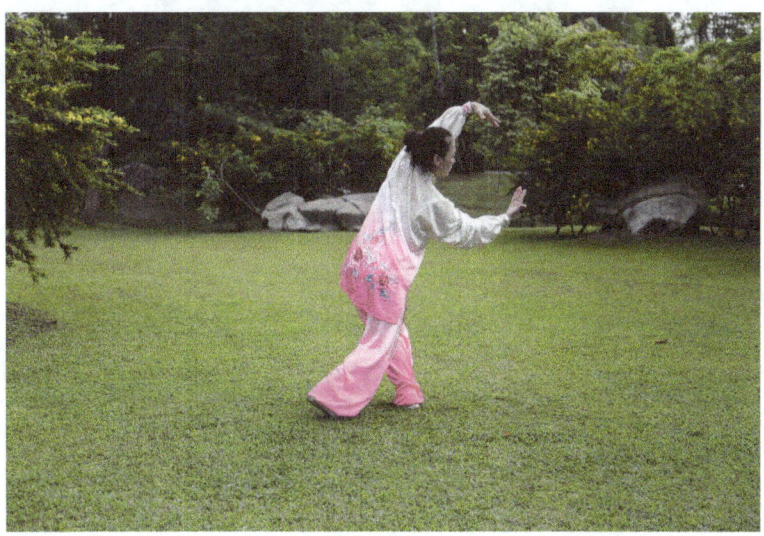

Fig. 6.88.

5. The right foot steps backward (west), while the upper body turns toward the right, with the two arms in a hugging posture, and continues to rotate to the right in an arc. Look at the space between the hands (Fig. 6.88).

Key Points

1. The form involves rotating two continuous rounds with the upper body, with the two arms in a hugging posture. The key is to perform it smoothly and continuously.
2. Both legs need to stay bent at the knee and keep the center of gravity stable. The two arms should stay in posture as if hugging a big ball and circle anti-clockwise vertically. When the hands roll up, the head leans back and the hip moves forward.
3. The form consists of two continuous rounds of circling. Beginners experiencing problems can perform one round instead.

29. Withdraw-step diverting palm

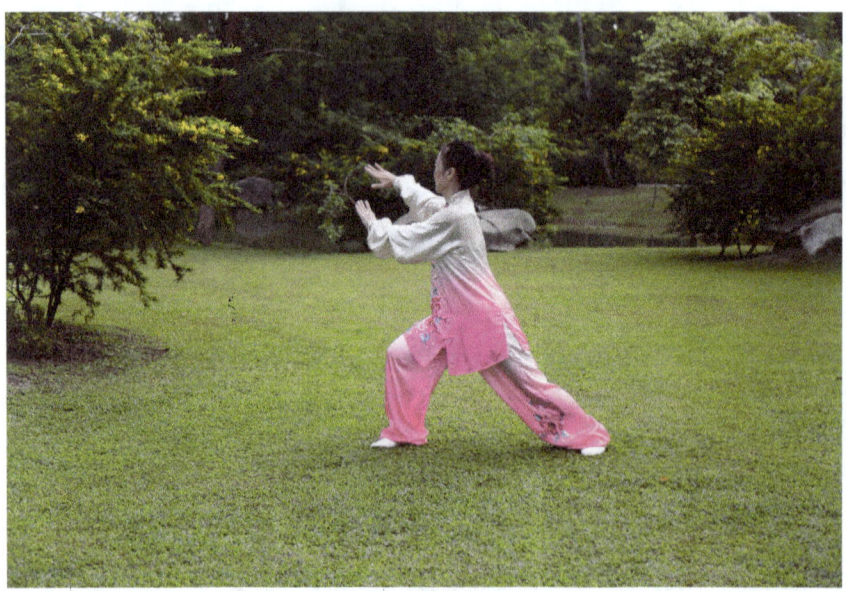

Fig. 6.89.

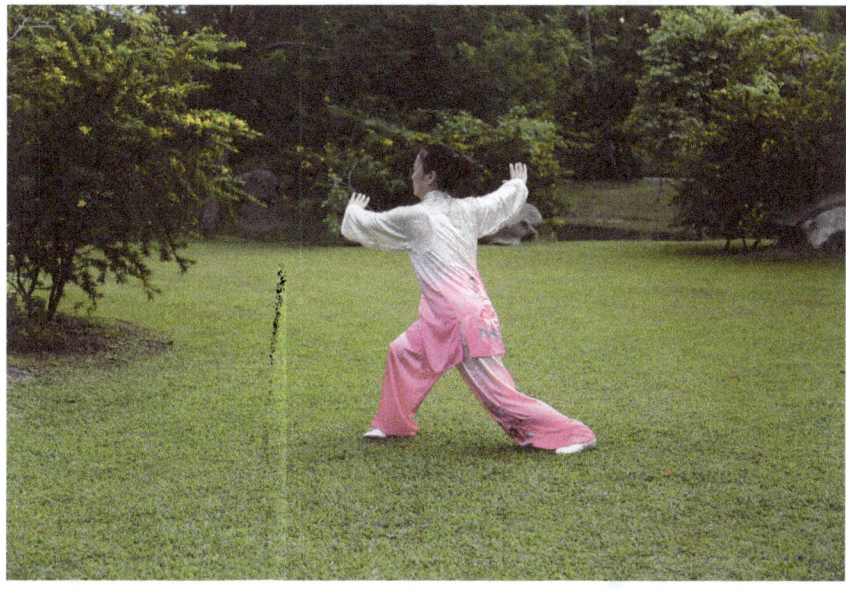

Fig. 6.90.

1. The body shifts rightward while turning right, the arms naturally swinging to the right back side horizontally and stretching straight with the momentum of the body spinning. The left arm bends slightly and the head turns right with it (Figs. 6.89 and 6.90).

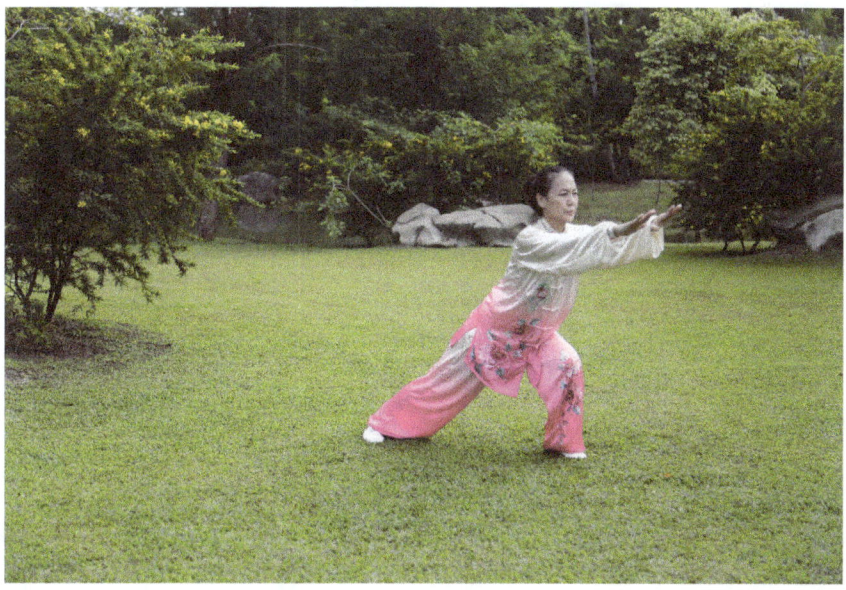

Fig. 6.91.

2. The body weight moves leftward while the upper body turns left. Keep the right leg close to straight, both arms swinging to the left in a horizontal circle with the body, arms extending straight, palms facing down, and look forward (Fig. 6.91).

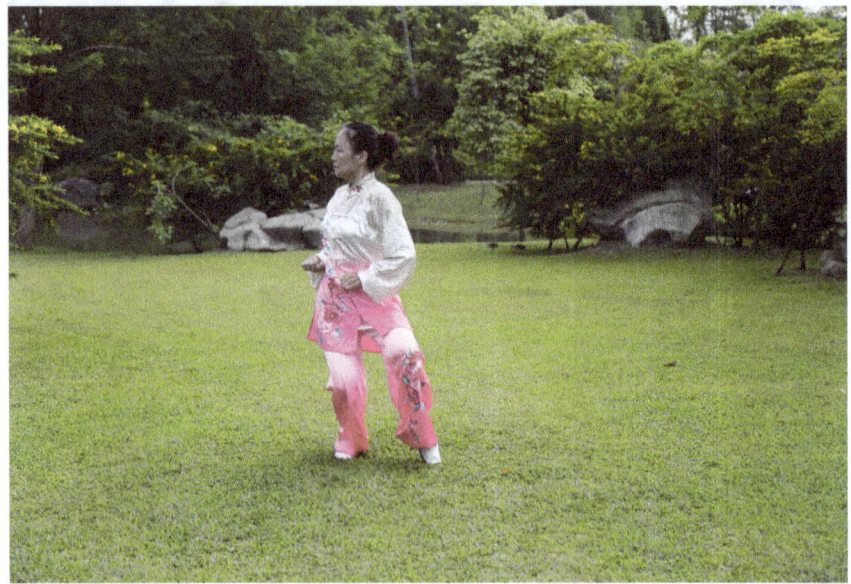

Fig. 6.92.

3. Push off with the left leg to move the center of gravity backward to the right leg, and turn right. The left foot withdraws back half a step and touches the ground with the toe only, both legs staying bent. At the same time, both arms withdraw quickly toward the waist with a pulling intention. This is called the shift palm. Then both hands turn to loosely formed fists with fingers bent, palms facing down. The head turns right at the same time (Fig. 6.92).

30. Forward-step pressing palm

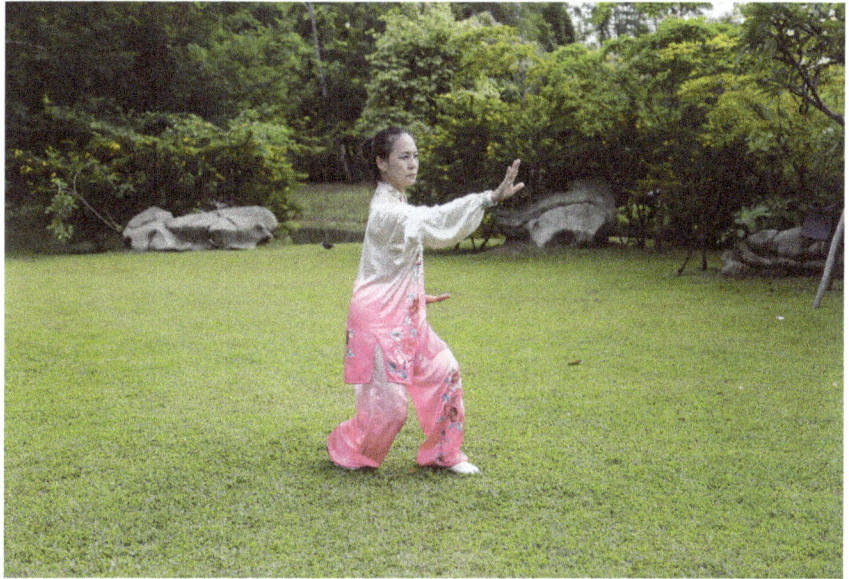

Fig. 6.93.

The body weight moves leftward gradually while the head and body turn gradually to the left. Next, the right leg pushes off, and the left foot steps forward quickly to the east. Then the right foot follows to move half a step forward and stops with the ball of the right foot touching the ground. Both legs bend with the center of gravity closer to the left foot. At the same time, the right hand changes to palm shape and pounces forward with wrist pressing downward and fingers kept apart, palms facing forward underneath. The left hand flexes flat before being placed over the left hip. Look to the right hand (Fig. 6.93).

Key Points

1. The pressing palm should be performed quickly and powerfully, with a power-restoring process before it releases.
2. The height of the pressing palm should be level with the chest or face depending on the target of attack.

31. Paring and wiping palm

Stop for a little while. Then turn the body slowly, slightly to the left, and swing the right arm slightly to the left. At the same time, the right hand rotates anti-clockwise to make the palm face up. Move the left palm gradually upward from above the left hip to the upper right side, while the body's center of gravity moves to the left completely.

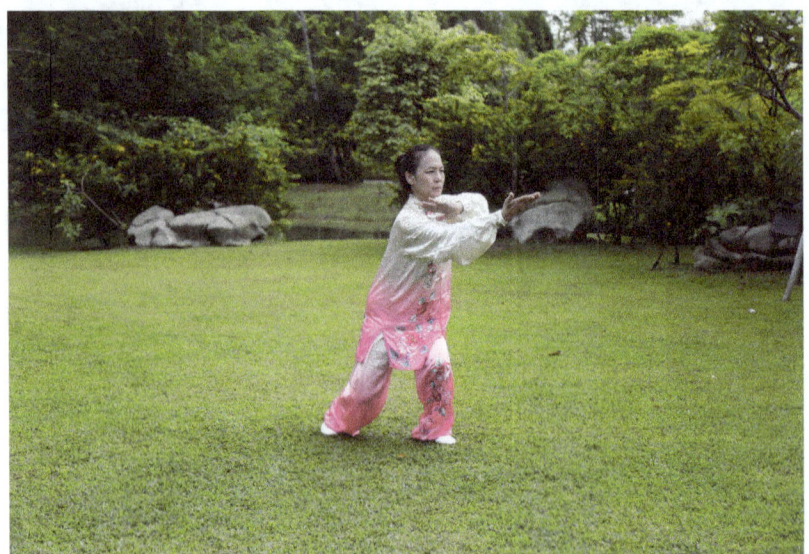

Fig. 6.94.

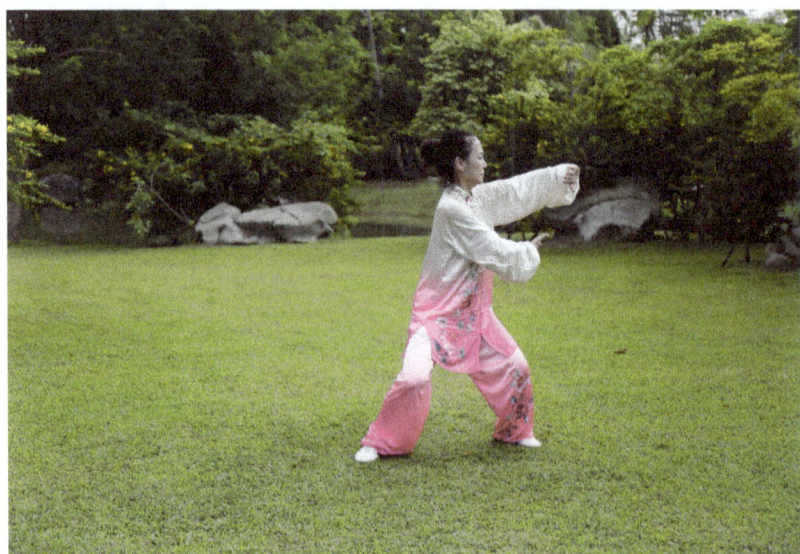

Fig. 6.95.

Next, the right foot moves to the right side for a small step, and the body quickly turns right (but only slightly in range), while the right palm moves quickly toward the back and lower right side in an arc, palm facing up. The left palm moves quickly along the right upper arm toward the right, forward, and left side in an arc, palm facing down. The right arm bends, and the left arm also bends slightly. Look to the left palm (Figs. 6.94 and 6.95).

Key Points

1. The slight left turn of the body at the beginning is a small transition action. It should be performed slowly but with an inner power and momentum ready to be released.
2. The right palm cuts and the left palm wipes. While performing, the left palm should be close above the right arm, and the right palm should be close under the left arm.

32. Side thrusting palm

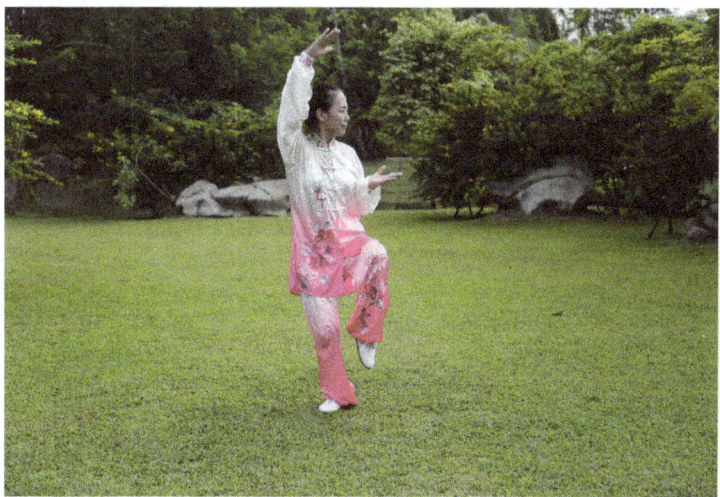

Fig. 6.96.

1. Continue from the previous form without stopping. The palms continue to move quickly toward the back and right side in an arc, while the center of gravity moves toward the right foot, with the right leg bent, left foot up. The right palm continuous to arc upward, palm facing to the lower left, with the left arm bent. The left palm withdraws, moving close to the chest in front while turning anti-clockwise to face up. Look to the left (Fig. 6.96).

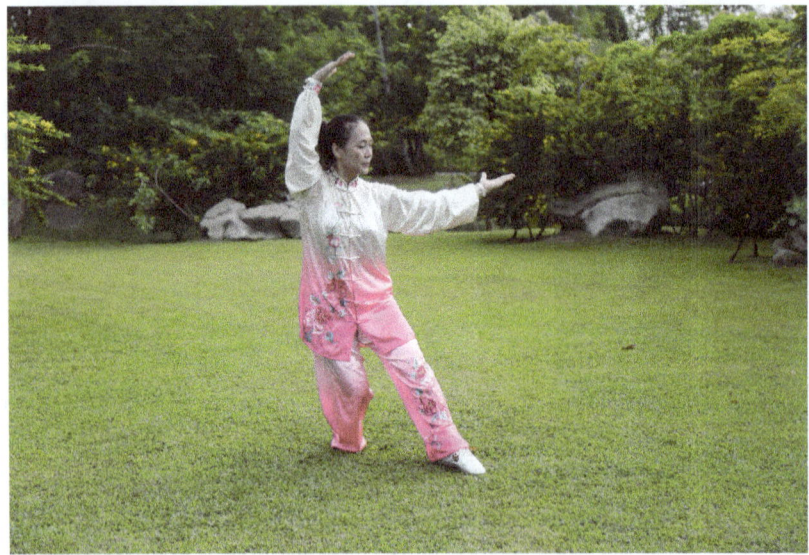

Fig. 6.97.

2. The left foot steps forward to the southeast, while the palms thrust to the left, with the right arm curved, right palm above the head and facing down. The left arm should be nearly straight, palm still facing up, with both hands keeping the fingers apart. Look toward the left palm (Fig. 6.97).

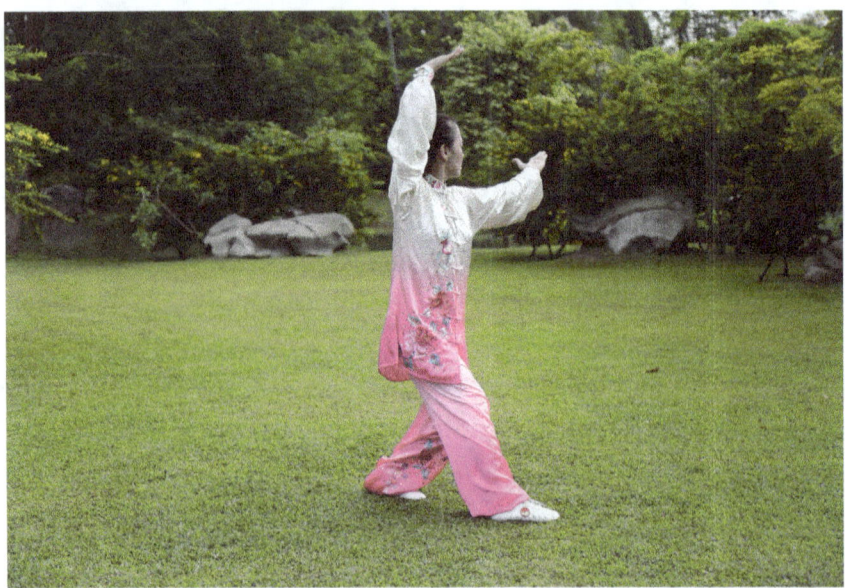

Fig. 6.98.

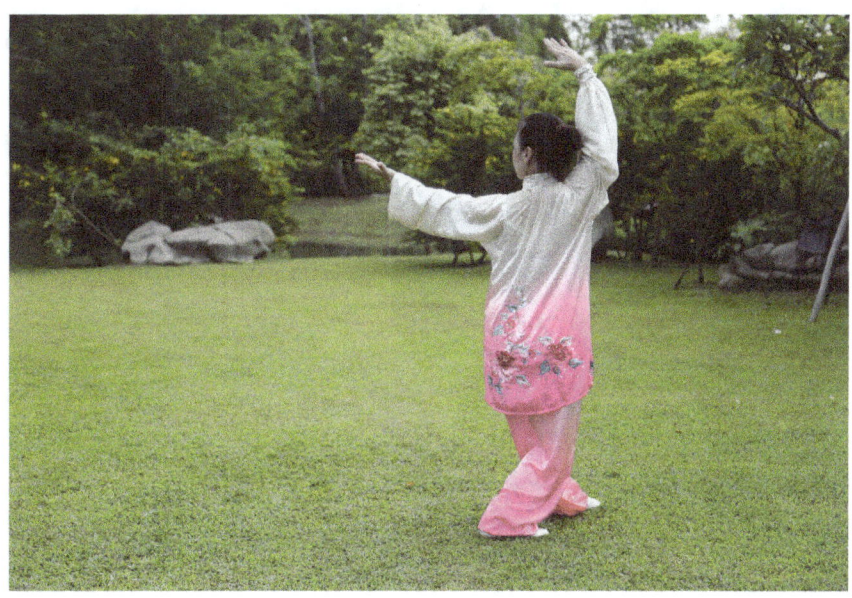

Fig. 6.99.

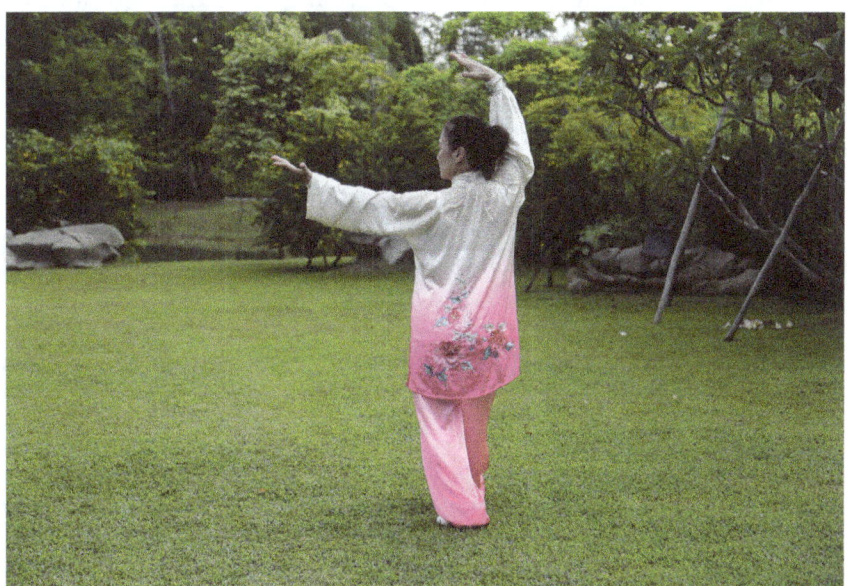

Fig. 6.100.

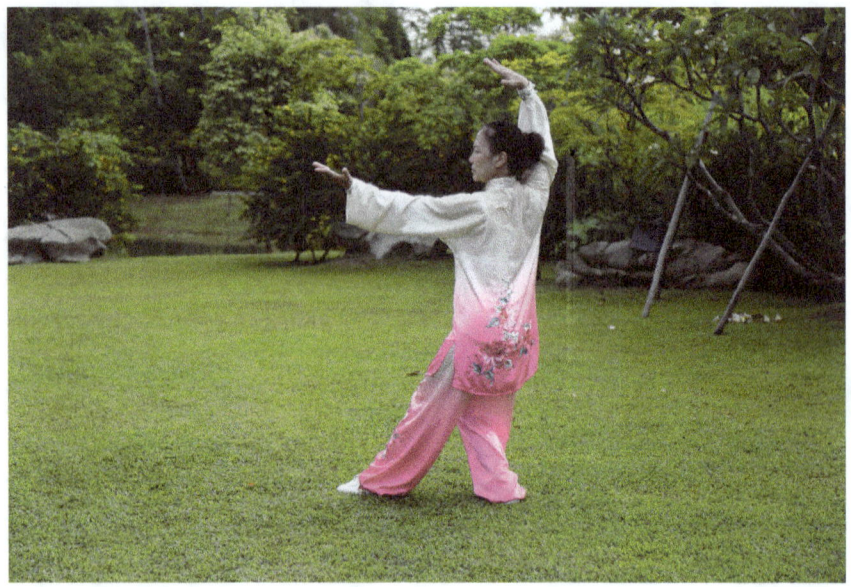

Fig. 6.101.

3. Continue with the last form without stopping, then the right foot wades toward the east, the left foot wades to the northeast, the right foot wades toward the north, and the left foot moves to the northwest; continues to wade four steps in an arc. The posture of the arms remains unchanged during the four steps. Always look to the left (Figs. 6.98–6.101).

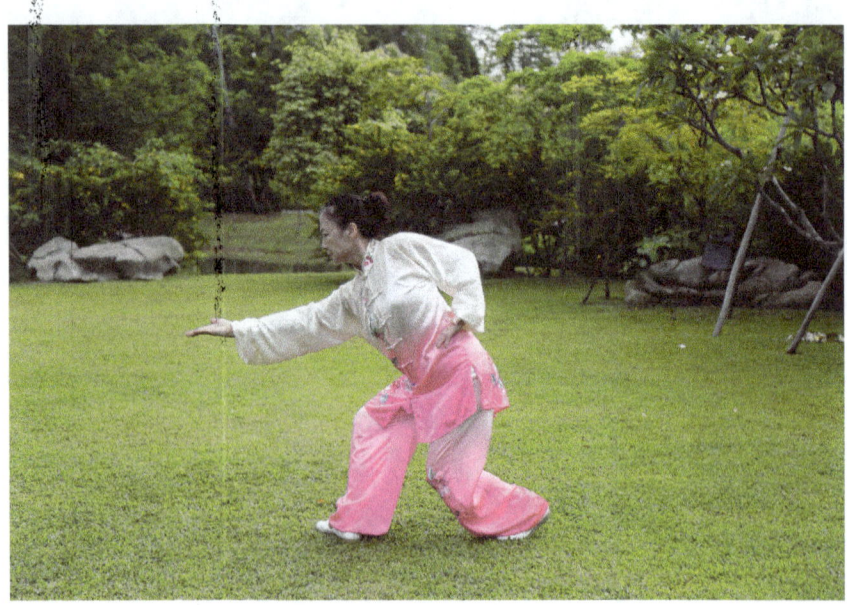

Fig. 6.102.

33. Forward-chopping palm

Step the right foot up to the northwest, and squat with the legs bent. At the same time, the right palm chops forward and down, palm facing up tilted, the fingers close together. Meanwhile, the left palm rapidly withdraws to the front right shoulder, palm facing up. Look at the right palm (Fig. 6.102).

34. Front cross-step chopping palm

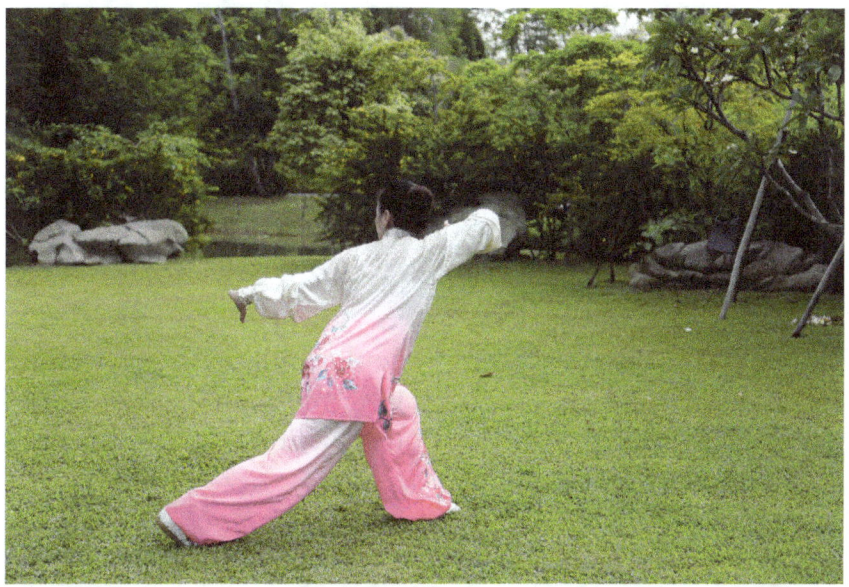

Fig. 6.103.

The left foot steps forward to cross over the right leg in an arc to the east (or northeast) direction. While the left foot is landing, the left palm quickly chops to the left and downward, palm facing down tilted. The power releasing point is at the outer edge of the palm. The right palm pulls back quickly to the front right shoulder, palm facing up. Look towards the left palm (Fig. 6.103).

35. Open stance rightward pairing palm

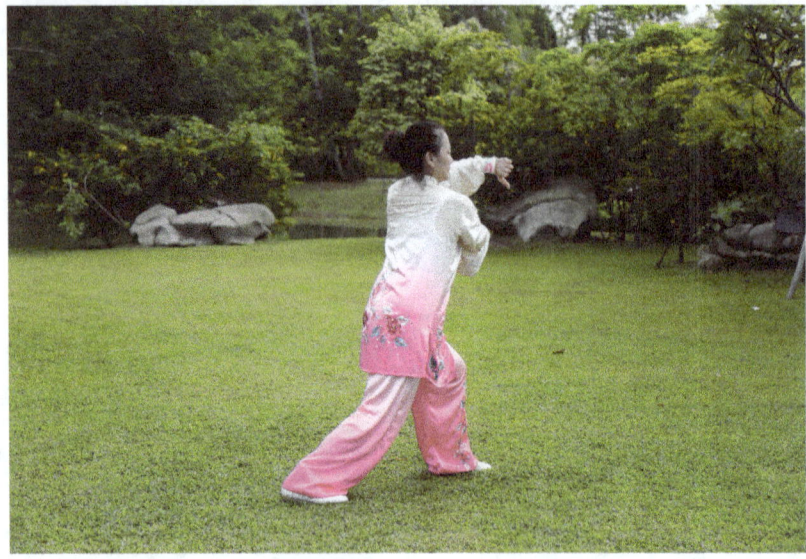

Fig. 6.104.

1. The body begins to turn right, while the left arm swings to the right and gradually bends, the left palm facing down. At the same time, the right palm pierces out from under the left armpit, palm still facing up (Fig. 6.104).

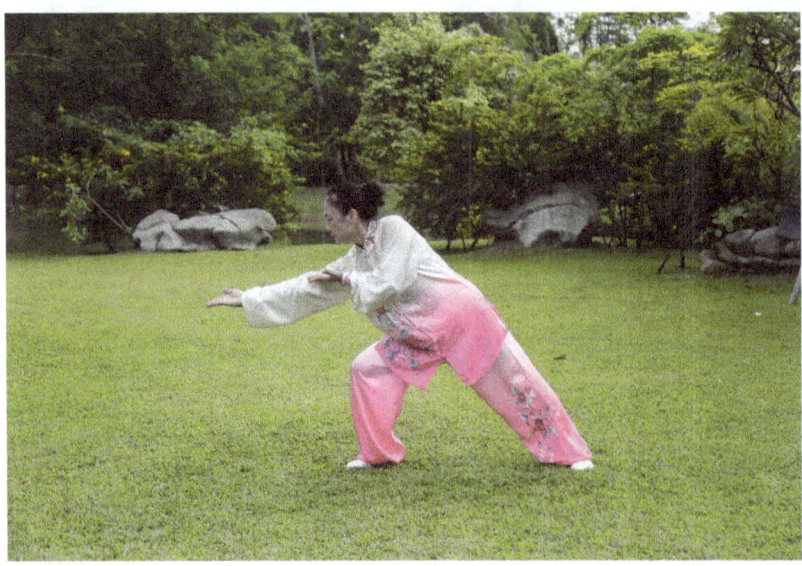

Fig. 6.105.

2. The body continues to turn right while the body weight moves to the right leg. The right palm continues to pierce from under the armpit, moving forward, to the right, and backward (west) to draw a large arc to complete a horizontal paring, palm facing up, with the upper body leaning slightly forward. At the same time, the left arm continues to bend and swing to the right. The left palm stops in front of the right shoulder. Look toward the right palm (Fig. 6.105).

Key Points

This form can be performed in a wide range, but not too fast or too fierce. Consciously, it can be treated as the preparation for the next form, which means that when this form has not been completed, the next form is visually constructed and ready to go.

36. Inward-latching step rotate body

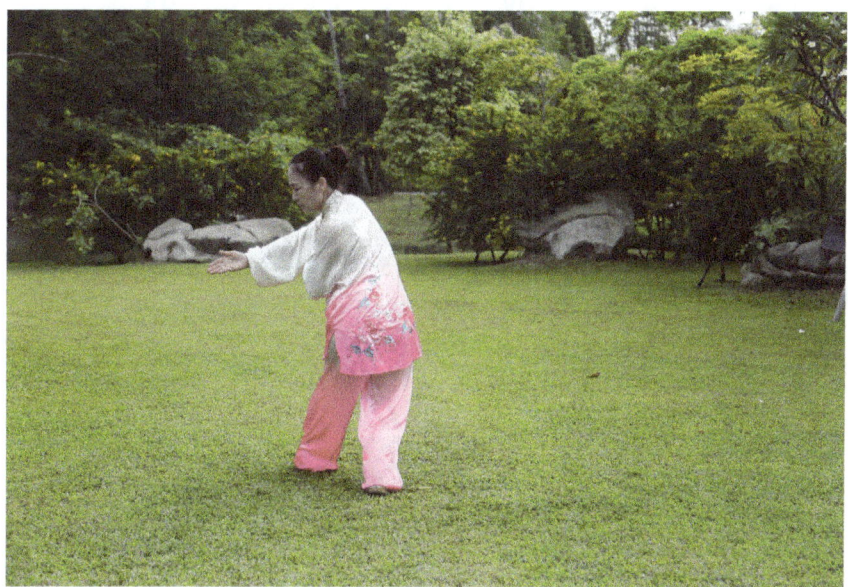

Fig. 6.106.

1. Without stopping, the left foot moves toward the right front (northwest) of the right foot to perform an inward-latching step (Fig. 6.106).

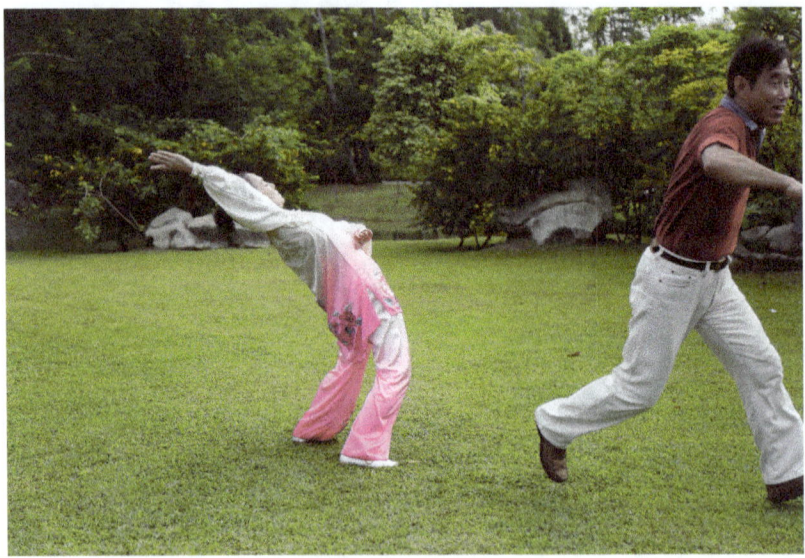

Fig. 6.107.

The upper body rolls to the right and leans back toward the west, sending the hips forward, while the right arm remains straight and points to the original direction, with the left palm placed under the right armpit, and the head thrown back (Fig. 6.107).

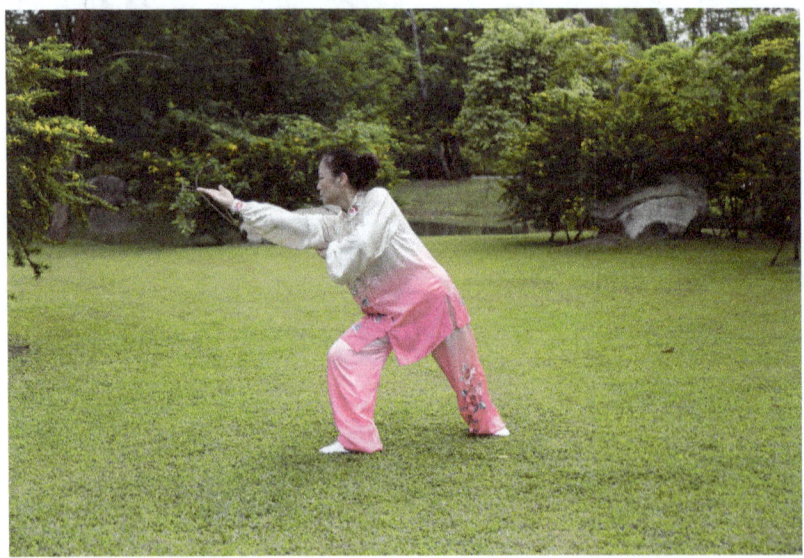

Fig. 6.108.

2. The upper body keeps rolling to the right, the right foot stepping to the west and facing west. The right arm remains straight and points to the west, with the left palm still placed under the right armpit (Fig. 6.108).

Key Points

1. The movement needs to be continuous and smooth, while the speed is decided by the individual situation.
2. The body rolling and turning should be like a rolling python, and the head and upper body should be as low as possible, but this should be decided according to each individual's flexibility — do not push yourself too hard.

37. Lean back kick with double thrusting palm

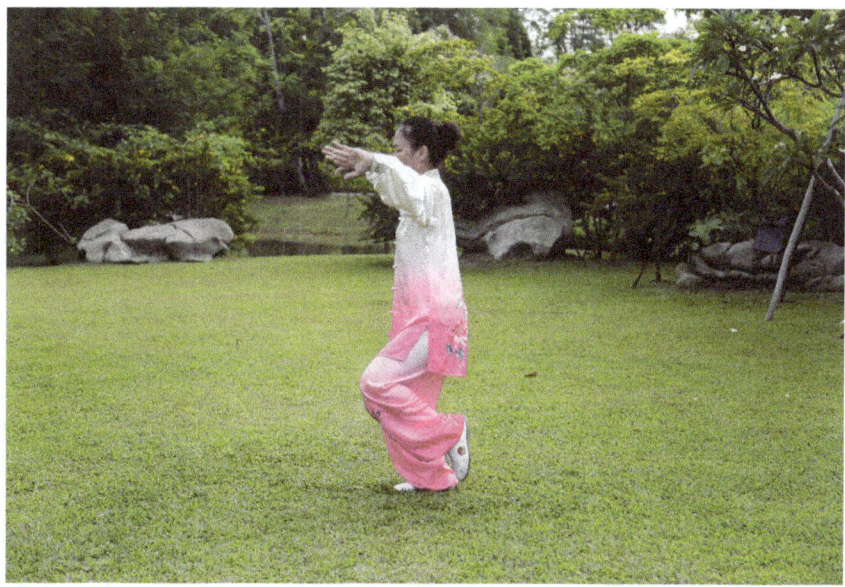

Fig. 6.109.

1. The left foot lifts up (west) and prepares to step forward, both hands swinging to the sides in an arc, with the arms slightly bent, palms facing outward and slightly above the shoulder (Fig. 6.109).

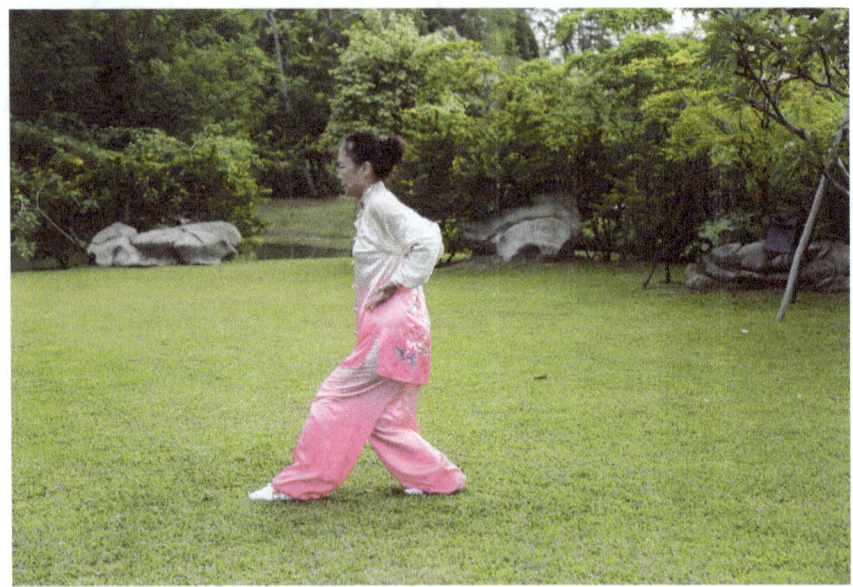

Fig. 6.110.

Next, the left foot lands forward and both palms withdraw to the waist. (Fig. 6.110).

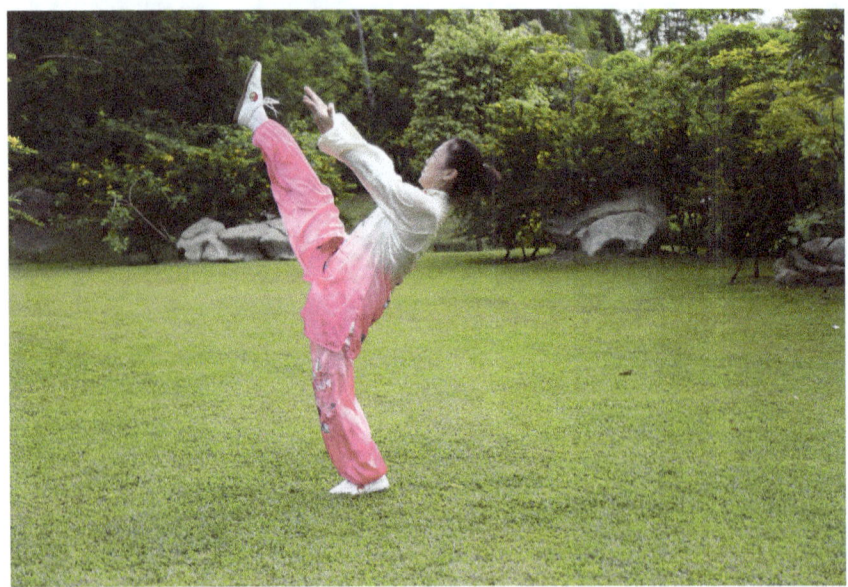

Fig. 6.111.

2. The right leg lifts up, bending, and then quickly kicks out toward the upper front until the leg is straight. The power releasing point is at the ball of the foot. At the same time, both palms thrust toward the upper front until the arms are straight. The upper body leans back slightly. Look toward the upper front (Fig. 6.111).

Key Points

While kicking, lift the right knee high and then quickly kick out, thrusting out the ball of the foot.

38. Crouching stance piercing palm

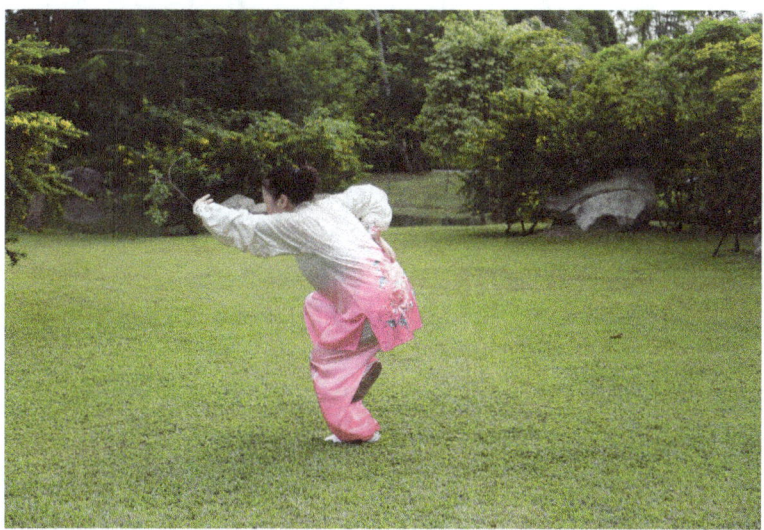

Fig. 6.112.

1. Rapidly withdraw the upper body and hold in the abdomen. The upper body turns back to an upright and slightly forward position, moving into a slightly forward posture from the lean-back position. The right foot lifts up and withdraws at the inner side of the left leg. The left leg bends and squats. At the same time, the right palm turns inward with the wrist bent, and the fingertips turn toward the left in a horizontal arc for half a circle, fingers pointing to the rear. The back of the palm touches the right waist close to the back, with the left arm slightly bent, and rotated anti-clockwise (Fig. 6.112).

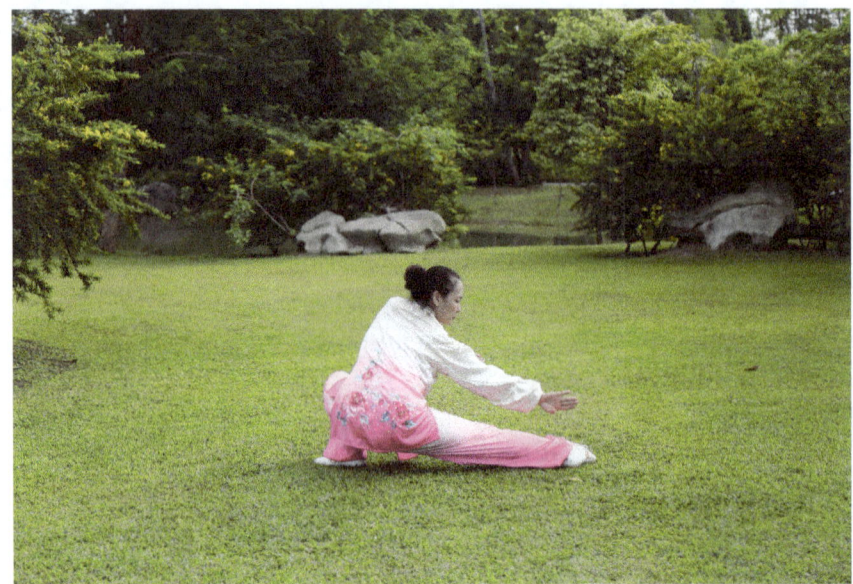

Fig. 6.113.

2. Bend the left leg to squat down fully while the right foot shovels to the east along the surface of the ground and lands with the right leg straight, the upper body turned slightly right to form the right crouching stance. At the same time, the right palm rotates clockwise to have the palm facing north and thrust out along the inside of the right leg toward the right foot. The left palm withdraws and stays in front of the belly. Look toward the right palm (Fig. 6.113).

Key Points

1. The crouching stance should stay low, with the hip and right leg as close to the ground as possible.
2. While beginning to withdraw the upper body and holding in the abdomen, the waist must be loosened. The upper body may turn left and right in a small range, so as to show a style like an undulating dragon. This requires delicate training and a good mastery of waist-loosening skill.

39. Heaven drilling palm with side-by-side foot stance

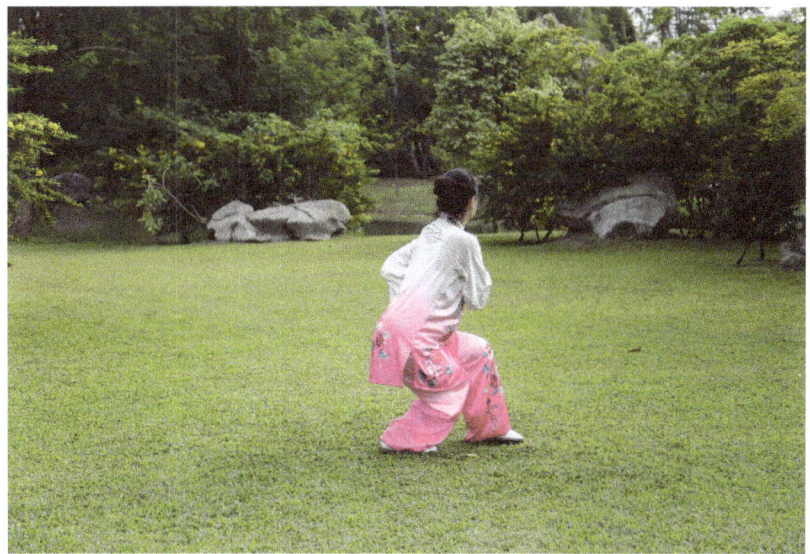

Fig. 6.114.

1. Without stopping, the center of gravity moves toward the right leg, while the left foot steps up to perform a small inward-latching step toward the east. Try to latch inward as much as possible, bending the legs and squatting down to keep a low posture. At the same time, the right arm folds, withdrawing the right palm to the chest (Fig. 6.114).

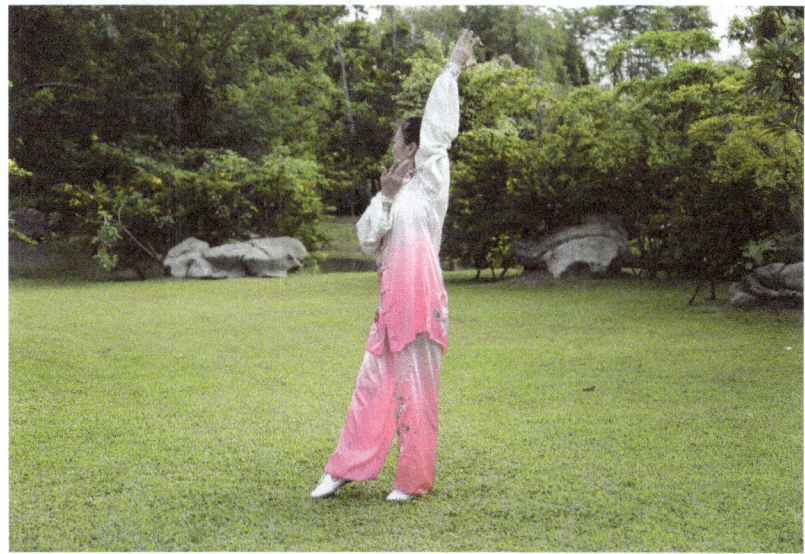

Fig. 6.115.

2. Push off with both legs to stand up gradually, keeping the body upright, and turn right. At the same time, the left palm thrusts out from under the right armpit and along the outside of the upper arm, rotating all the way clockwise, as if trying to drill a hole into the sky, palm facing backward when completed. Along the inside of the left arm, the right palm falls to the chest, rotating as much as possible anti-clockwise, palm facing rightward, holding the fingertips upward (Fig. 6.115).

Key Points

Try to practice with a personal rhythm and style. It could be done fast, but it will be perfect if the unique inner power and charm of this form can be expressed through the gradual standing up of the body and the gradual drilling up of the left palm while turning right. This demands that the practitioner personally appreciate the art, which will then lead to final enlightenment.

40. Tuck-in and left-and-right bumping palm

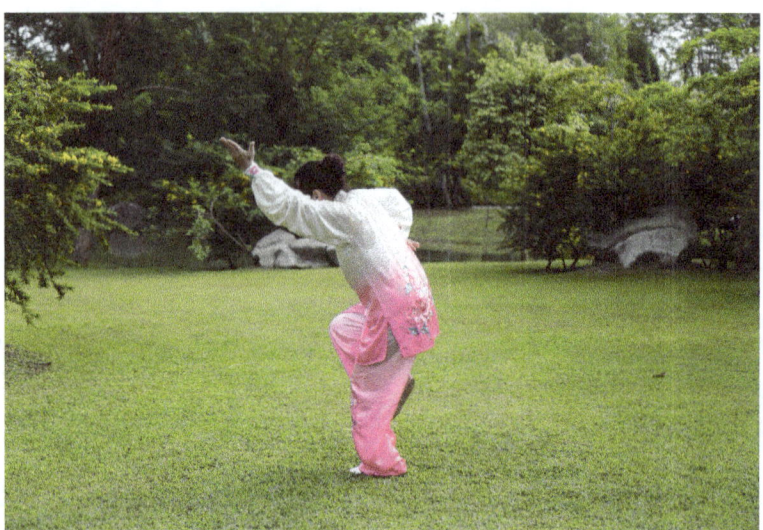

Fig. 6.116.

1. The body keeps turning right, while the left leg bends to squat down. Lift up the right foot, and fold the right arm with the wrist twisting in an inward spiral to have the back side of the fingers passing close to the chest, and then sliding to the right waist, the outer edge of the right palm facing up tilted. The right arm bends, and the left arm starts to drop to the left (Fig. 6.116).

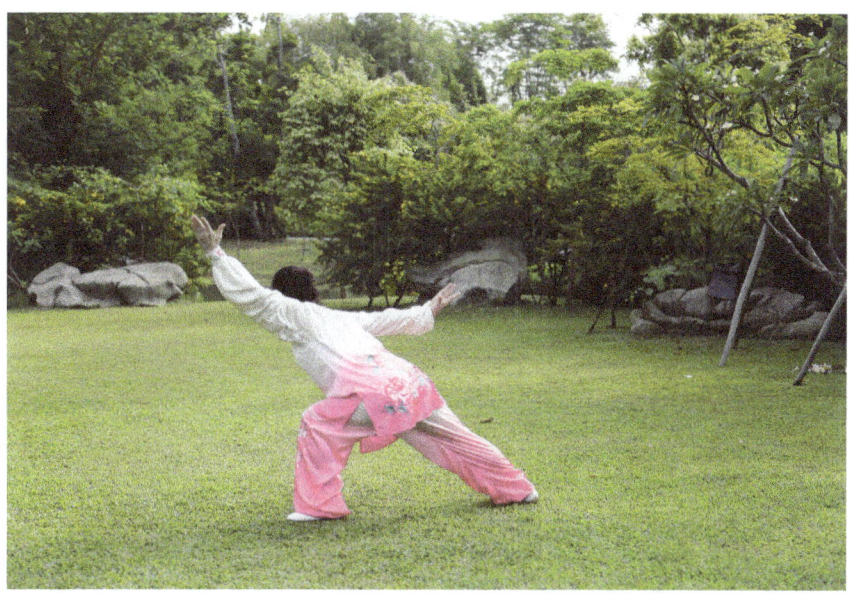

Fig. 6.117.

2. The right foot strides to the west, and the right palm thrusts out toward the right, palm facing up (Fig. 6.117).

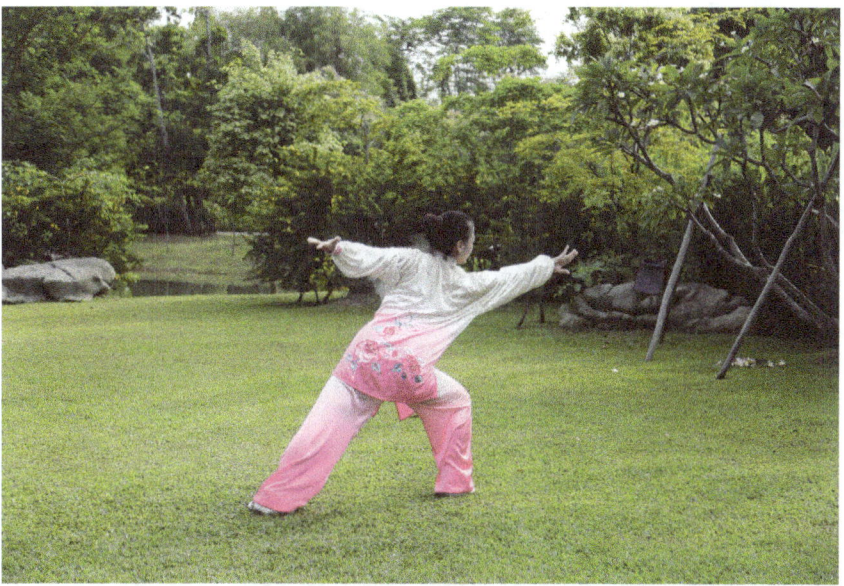

Fig. 6.118.

Without stopping, the left leg pushes off to shift the body weight rightward, and the right palm keeps reaching far and turns clockwise. Look toward the right hand (Fig. 6.118).

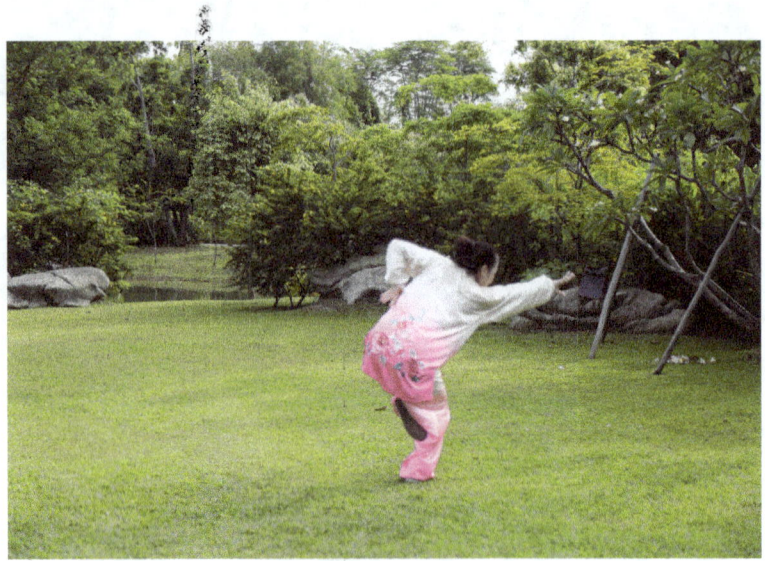

Fig. 6.119.

3. The left palm withdraws to the left waist, turning clockwise to make the back side of the palm touch the back near the waist, fingers pointing left. At the same time, lift up the left foot and keep looking toward the right (Fig. 6.119).

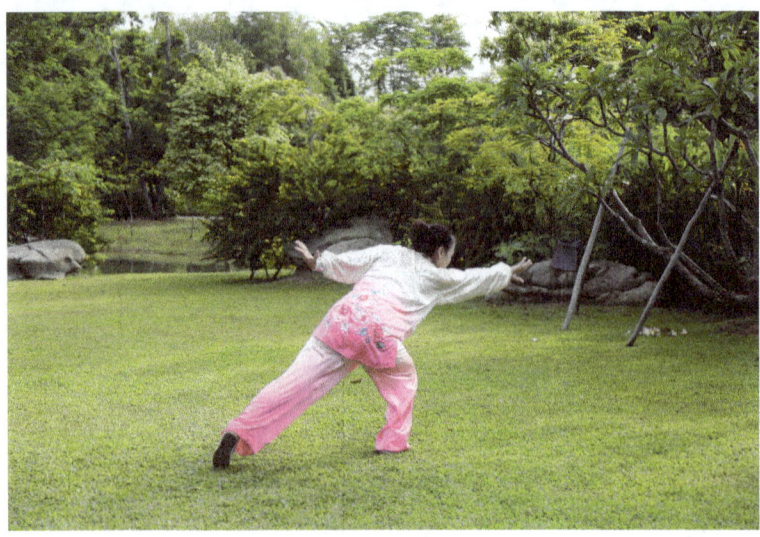

Fig. 6.120.

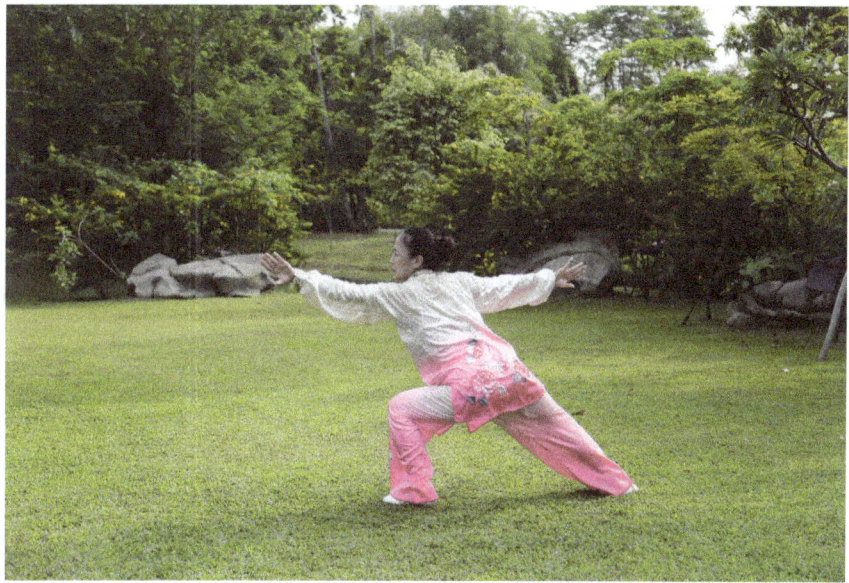

Fig. 6.121.

4. The left foot strides to the left while the body weight is shifted toward the left, and the left palm thrust leftward (Figs. 6.120 and Fig. 6.121).

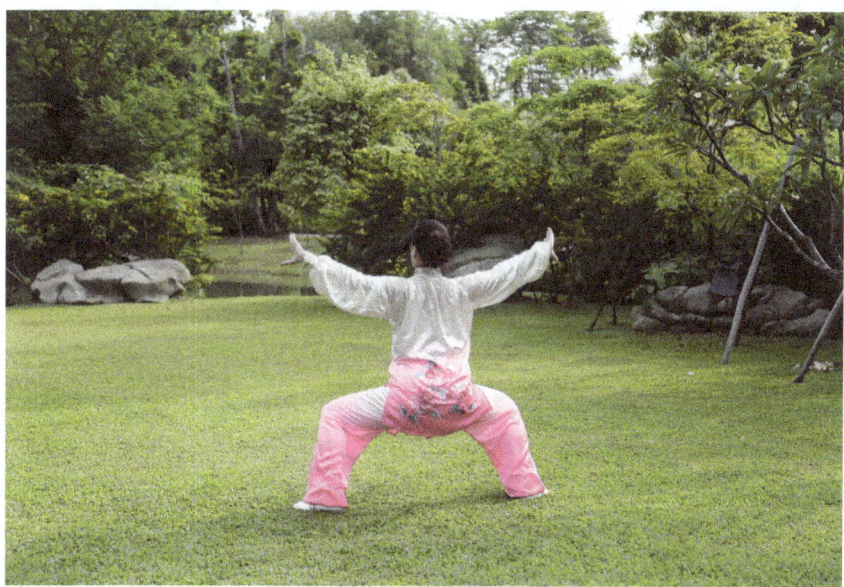

Fig. 6.122.

5. The center of gravity comes back in between the legs and shifts to the left and then right, with the palms fast and powerful but moving in a small range (Fig. 6.122).

Key Points

1. Steps 1–4 do not need to be performed too fast, but both the body movement and the thrust of the palms need to be done with significant range. The movement should be flexible but performed with inner power.
2. Step 5 should be of small range but very fast and powerful. It is almost like a shivering of the whole body toward the left and right, but the upper body needs to be upright while maintaining a powerful feeling inside. There could be a stop after the form is completed, but the powerful stance should remain.

41. Outward-swing and inward-latching steps and cloudy palm

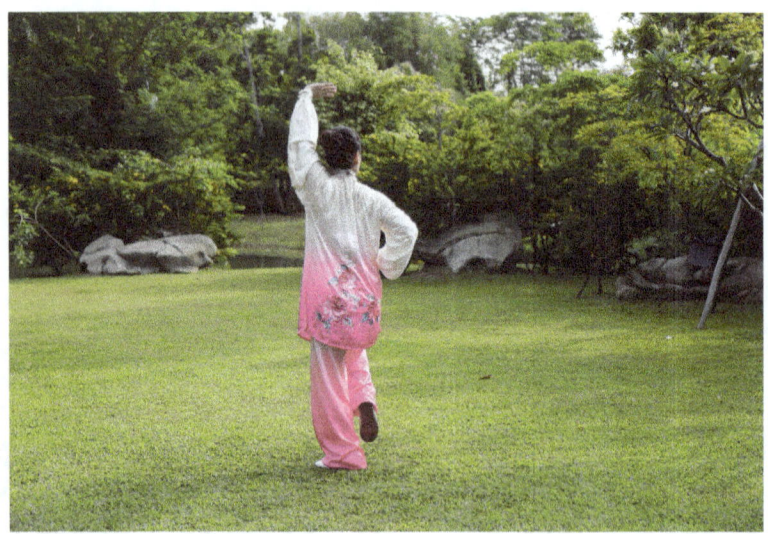

Fig. 6.123.

1. The body weight moves onto the left leg, which is kept bent, while the right foot lifts up and steps forward along the inside of the left foot. At the same time, the left palm lifts up, forming a block above the head, and the right arm bends to withdraw the right palm to the right waist, palm facing up (Fig. 6.123).

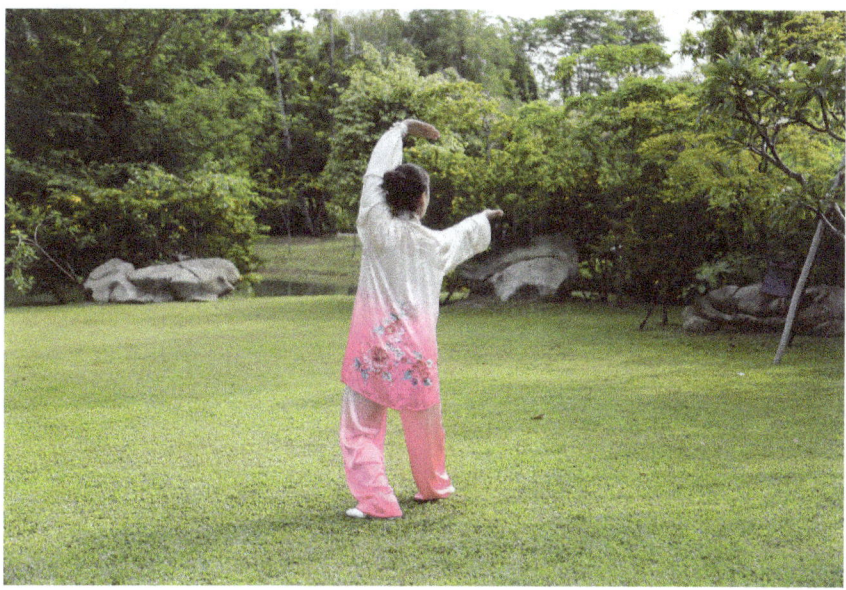

Fig. 6.124.

2. At the same time, the right palm waves in an arc toward the left and then the upper right (Fig. 6.124).

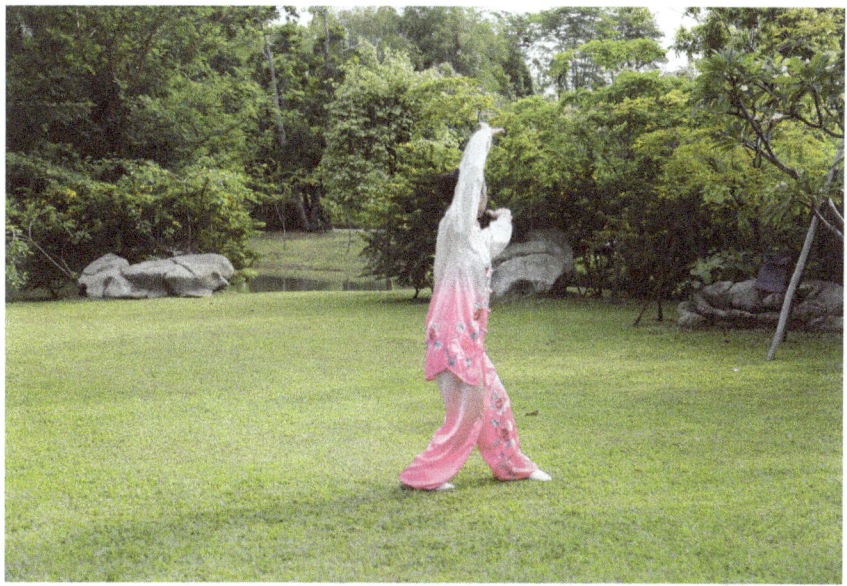

Fig. 6.125.

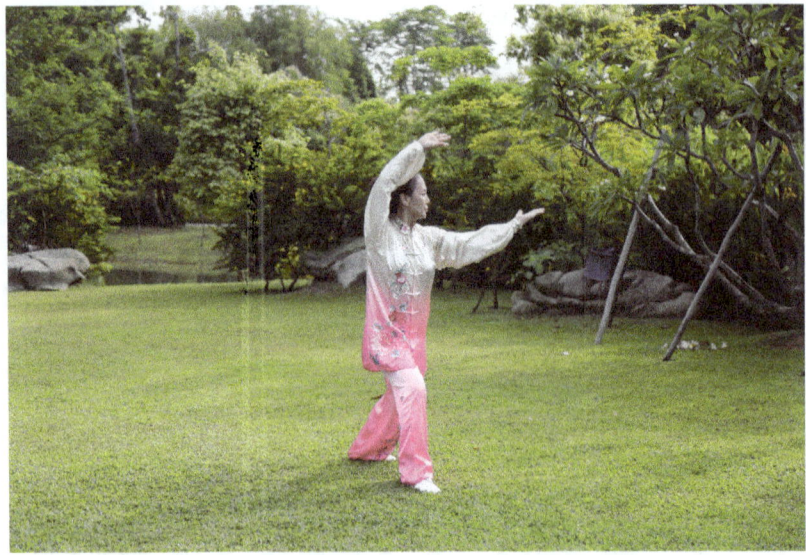

Fig. 6.126.

The left foot performs an inward-latching step toward the northeast, and then the right foot performs an outward-swing step toward the southeast. At the same time, the palms perform the cloudy palms above the head by waving in a circle clockwise to the right (Figs. 6.125 and 6.126).

42. Horizontal opening chop with a turn

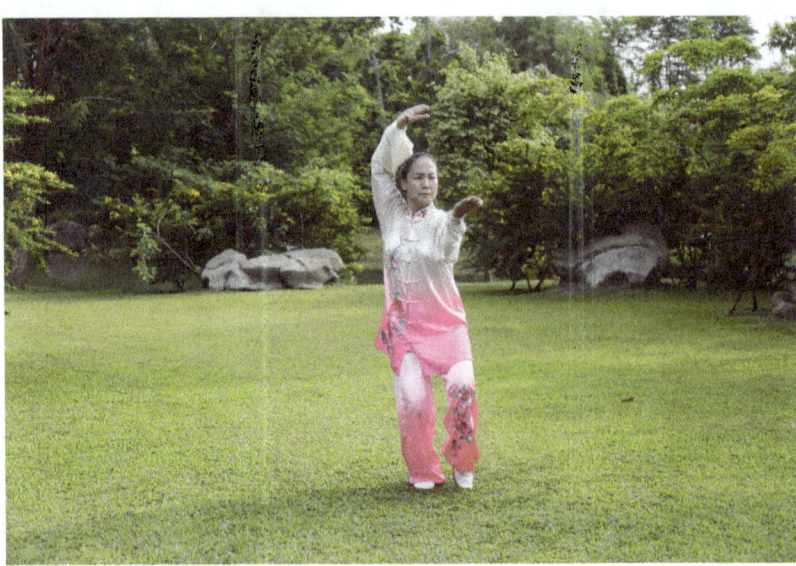

Fig. 6.127.

The left foot steps up toward the inside of the right foot, toes touching the ground without much force and with the legs bent, while the upper body turns right and releases power in a very short time, driving the left palm to chop horizontally toward the right side in front of the body, palm facing up. The power release point is in the outer edge of the left hand, at a height of about chest level, the right palm held above the head. Look toward the south in the direction of the left hand (straight ahead) (Fig. 6.127).

Key Points

The power release should be short and strong. There should be a bouncing-back potential toward the left after the powerful chopping to the right.

43. Left stride tuck-in and bumping palm

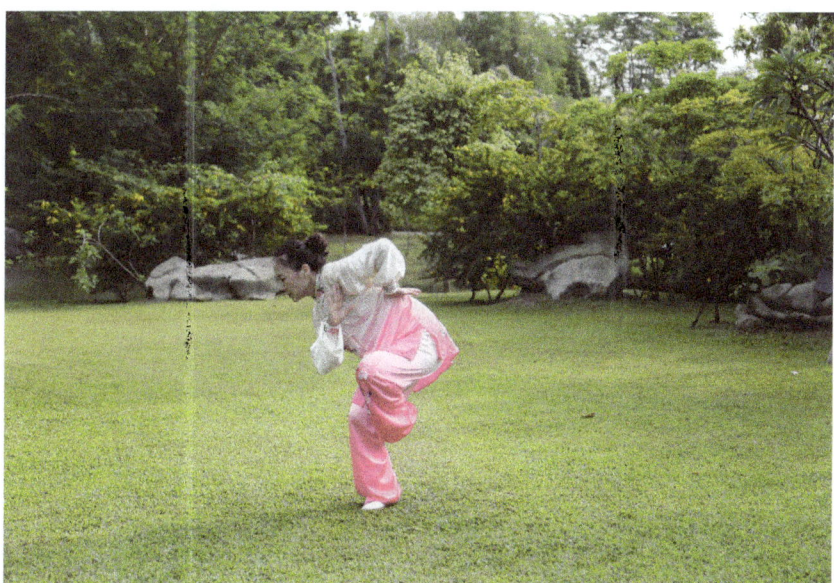

Fig. 6.128.

1. The left foot lifts up, while the upper body withdraws and leans toward the right. At the same time, the left arm folds with the wrist twisting to stay at the left ribs, the left palm facing up, fingers pointing to the left (Fig. 6.128).

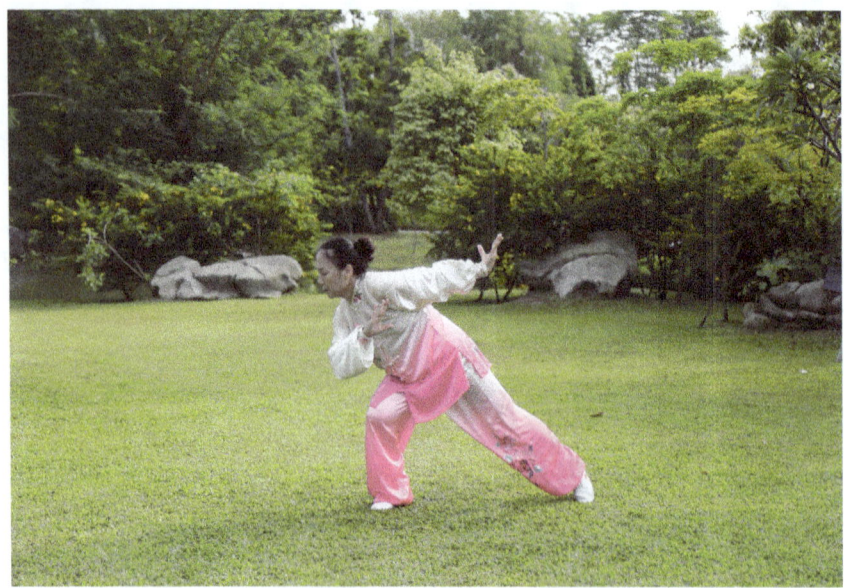

Fig. 6.129.

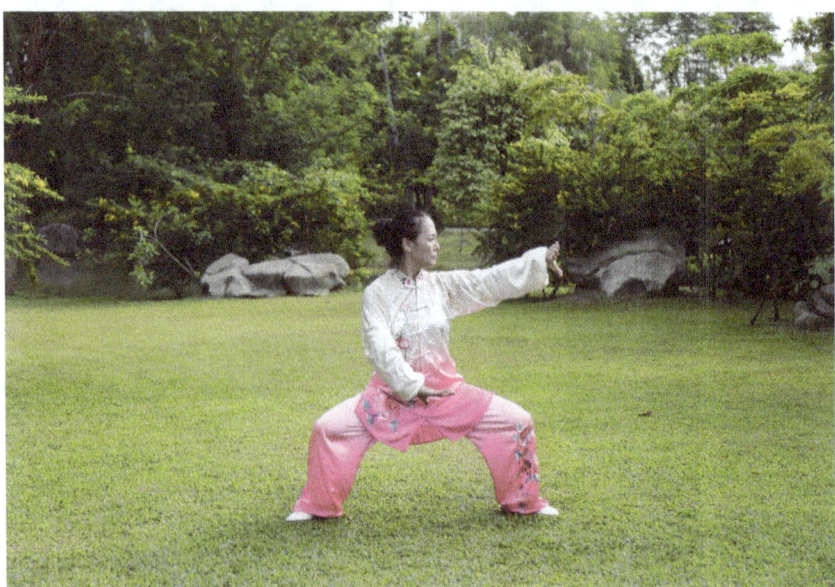

Fig. 6.130.

2. The left foot strides to the left and the left palm tucks in and thrusts out toward the left, while the body's center of gravity moves left in between

the legs. The left arm keeps on stretching further until it is straight, palm facing outside to continue to bump. The right palm pushes down in front the body, Look in the direction of the left palm (Figs. 6.129 and 6.130).

The tuck-in should be followed by bumping palm, without stopping (use palm to hit, not with movement of the arm, but with movement of the body, while keeping the arm straight).

44. Join up and tuck-in leftward opening palm

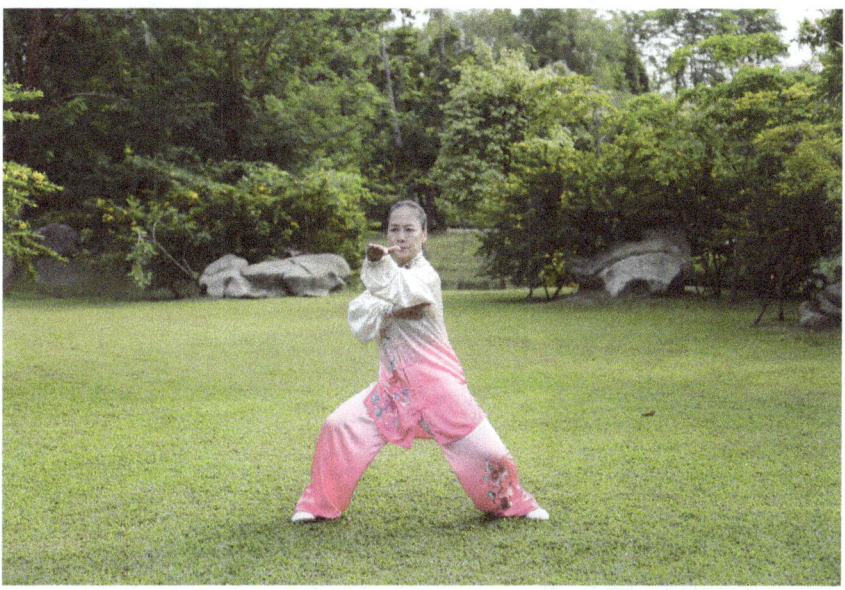

Fig. 6.131.

1. Turn right, the left arm swinging to the right horizontally and staying in front of the body, while the left palm rotates anti-clockwise to face up. The right palm is raised to the chest and rotates clockwise to face down (Fig. 6.131).

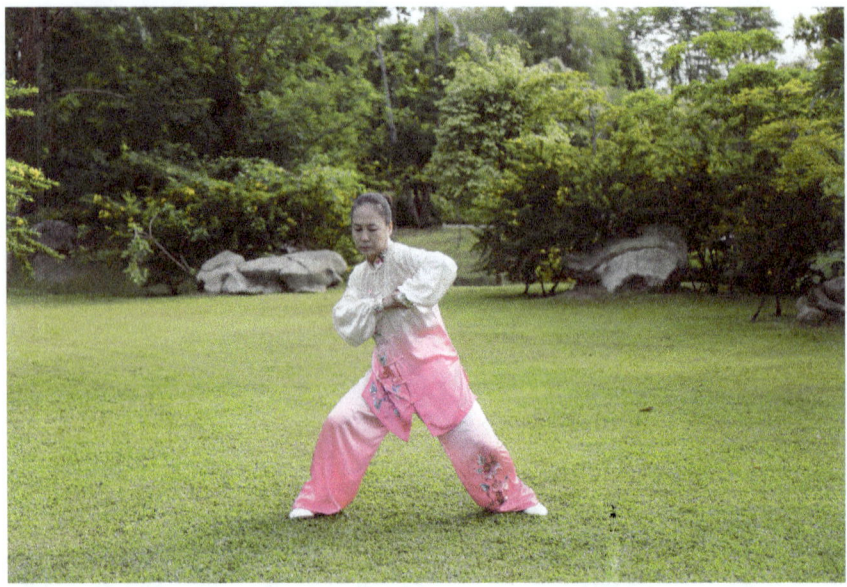

Fig. 6.132.

2. The left arm bends, and the left palm turns clockwise to twist the wrist and withdraw the palm to the left waist, to prepare for the backward tuck-in palm. The body weight moves toward the right (Fig. 6.132).

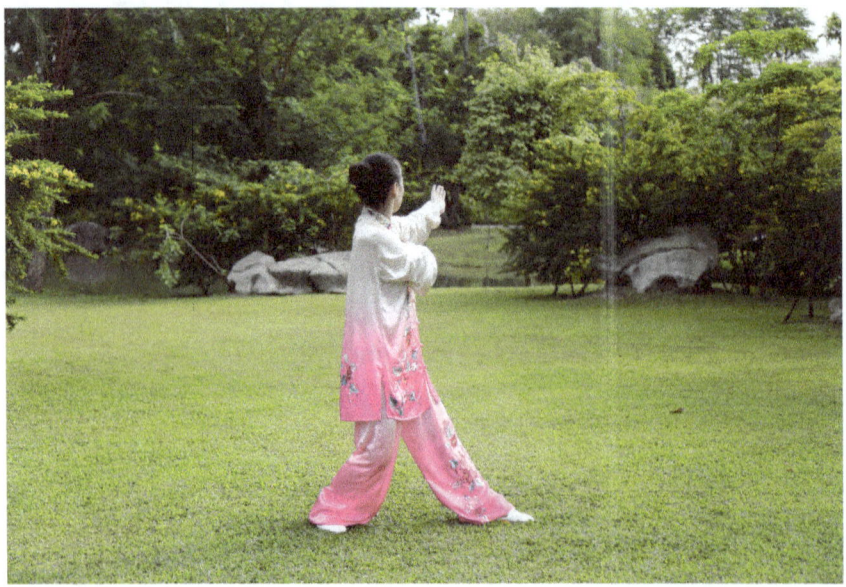

Fig. 6.133.

The left foot strides backward to the left, and the left palm thrusts out backward. The body turns left, and the right palm prepares to thrust out from under the left armpit, and the head turns left (Fig. 6.133).

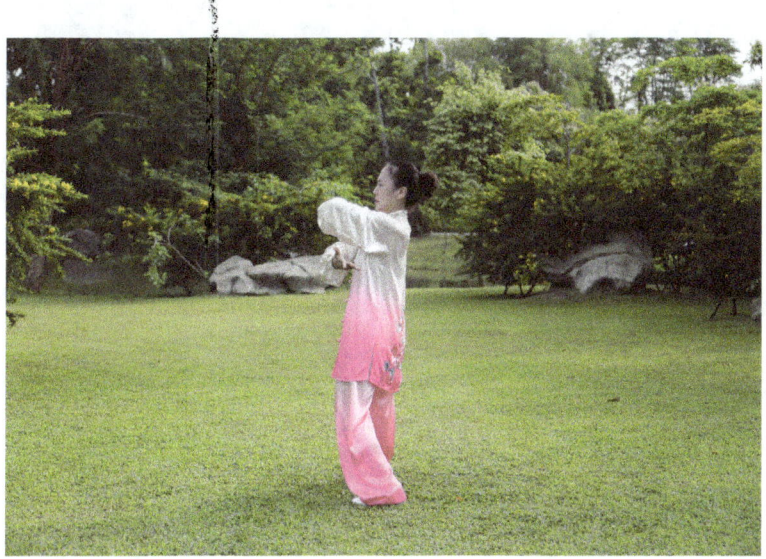

Fig. 6.134.

3. The body keeps turning left, while the right foot steps up northward. The right palm thrusts out from under the left armpit, and the left arm bends to form an arc. The head turns left (Fig. 6.134).

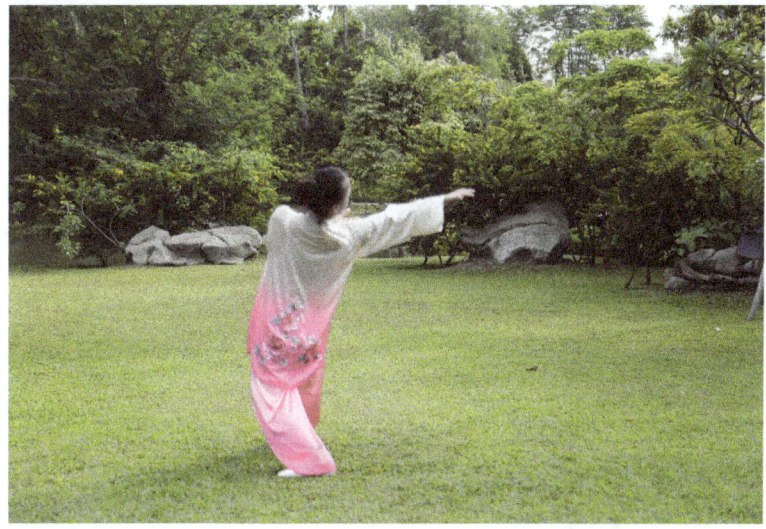

Fig. 6.135a.

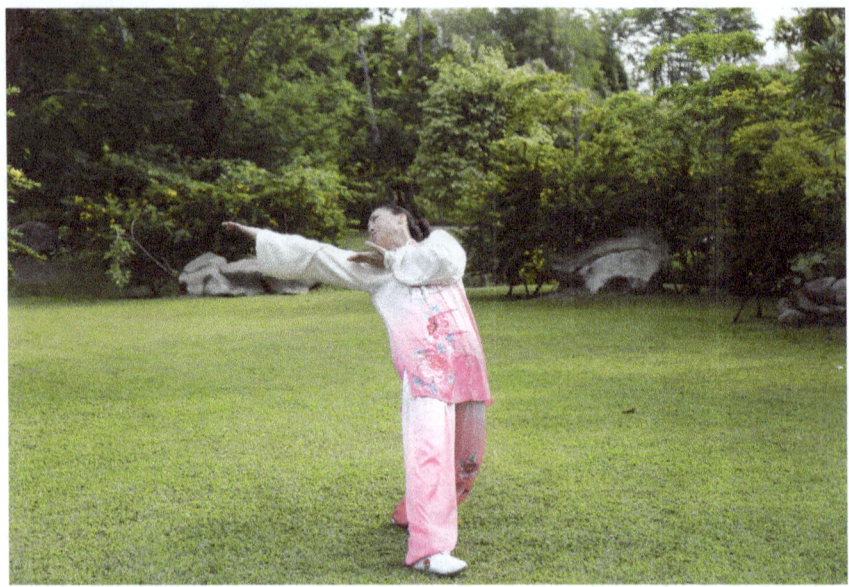

Fig. 6.135b.

4. The upper body leans back, with the left leg bent and the center of gravity staying on the left leg. The right leg stretches straight, and the right toe touches the ground. At the same time, the right palm swings horizontally from along the lower left arm to the left, front, and right until pointing to the east. The left palm swings along the right arm to the right, and arcs backward to reach the right shoulder, palm facing up, chest facing the north. Look at the right palm (Figs. 6.135a and 6.135b).

Key Points

Be fast and coherent when performing all these forms (except the movement shown in Fig. 6.135 a & b), which is the lean body opening palm. It should be performed slowly but with a big range.

45. Right drilling palm

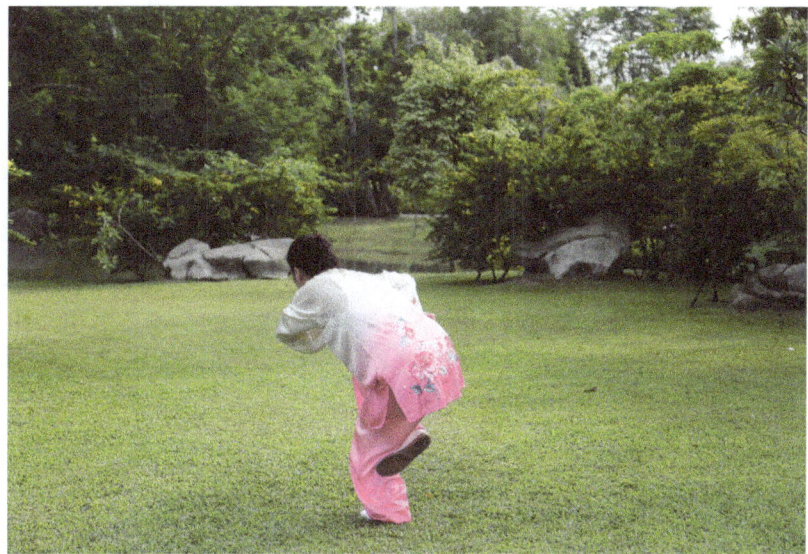

Fig. 6.136.

1. Rapidly lift up the right foot and withdraw it at the inner side of the left knee. Withdraw the upper body and hold in the abdomen, while the upper body leans left. At the same time, the right arm bends quickly and the right palm turns inward with the wrist bent near the right ribs, and the fingertips pointing to the right (Fig. 6.136).

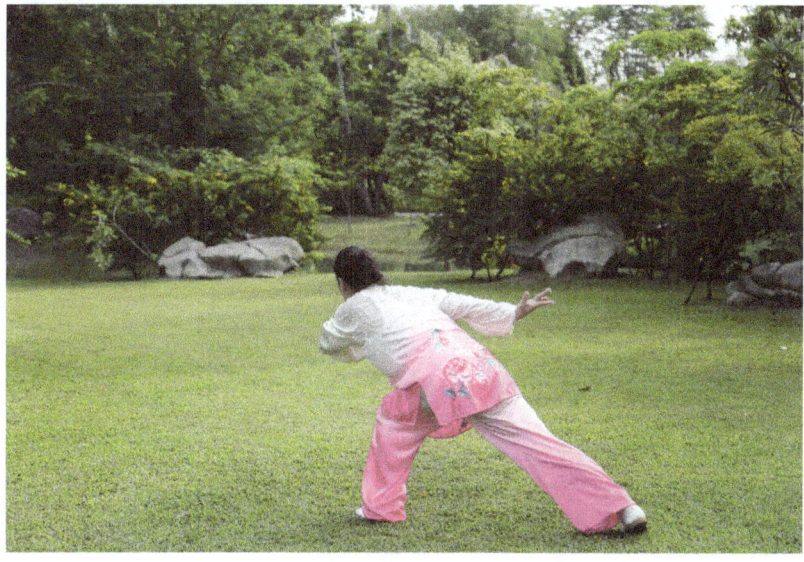

Fig. 6.137.

2. The right foot strides to the right, and the right palm drills out horizontally toward the right (Fig. 6.137).

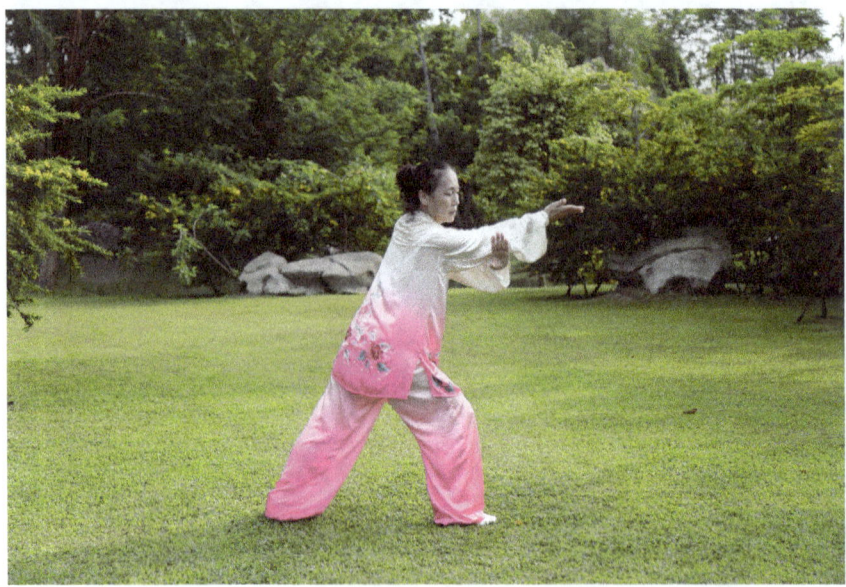

Fig. 6.138.

Push off with the left leg to move the center of gravity rightward quickly, and turn right. At the same time, the right palm keeps drilling toward the right, and the right arm extends straight naturally. The left hand slips below the right upper arm and starts to push forward with stand-up palm. Gaze toward the right hand (east) (Fig. 6.138).

46. Windmill-style chopping palm

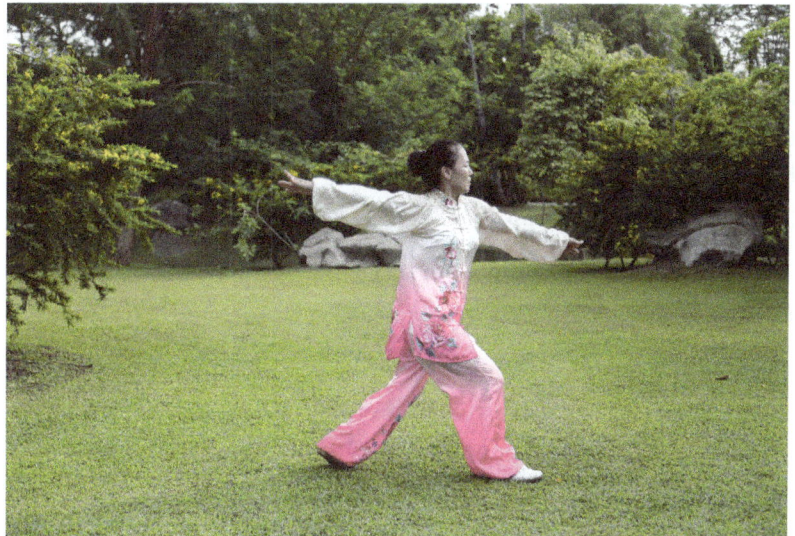

Fig. 6.139.

1. Continue from the previous form without stopping. Move forward and turn right. The left foot steps forward, and the left palm pushes forward at the same time, straightening the left arm. The right arm bends, and the right palm pulls back to slap toward the back side (west). The right arm is naturally pulled straight (Fig. 6.139).

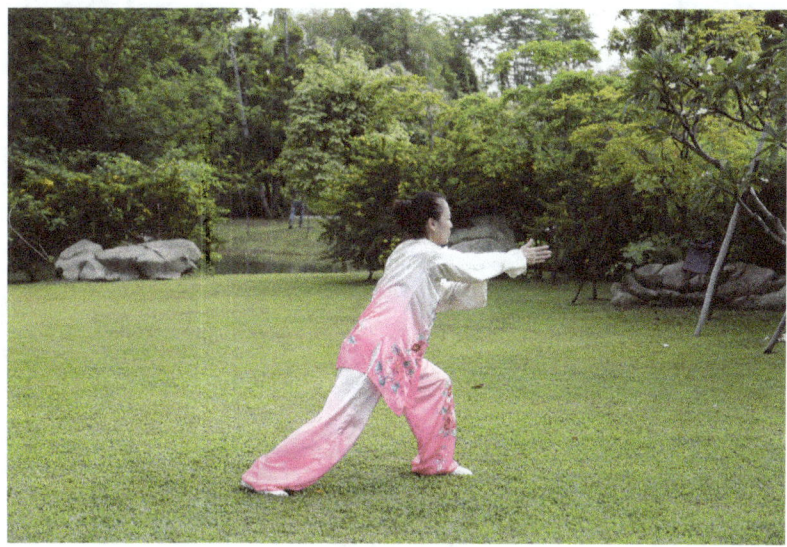

Fig. 6.140.

2. The left foot steps forward and the body weight moves forward, while the left leg bends and the right leg pushes off straight and forms a left bow stance. At the same time, the right palm keeps swinging in a round circle from above the head, moving forward and then chopping down. The right arm stays straight, with the height of the right palm leveled with the shoulder, palm facing left, and the palm edge pointing down. While the right palm chops down, the left palm rubs with the inner side of the right forearm with a clap (Fig. 6.140).

Key Points

1. Perform this form continuously without stopping. The timing of the left foot stepping forward should be flexible and tuned to personal habits. Focus on the footwork and arm swinging. The chopping of the palm should be a coordinated effort in favor of the individual power-releasing action.
2. This form is a whole vertical round swing for the right arm. The swing and chopping should be of great momentum, not just physically, but also with inner mindfulness, which is very important.

47. Lifting and bumping palm

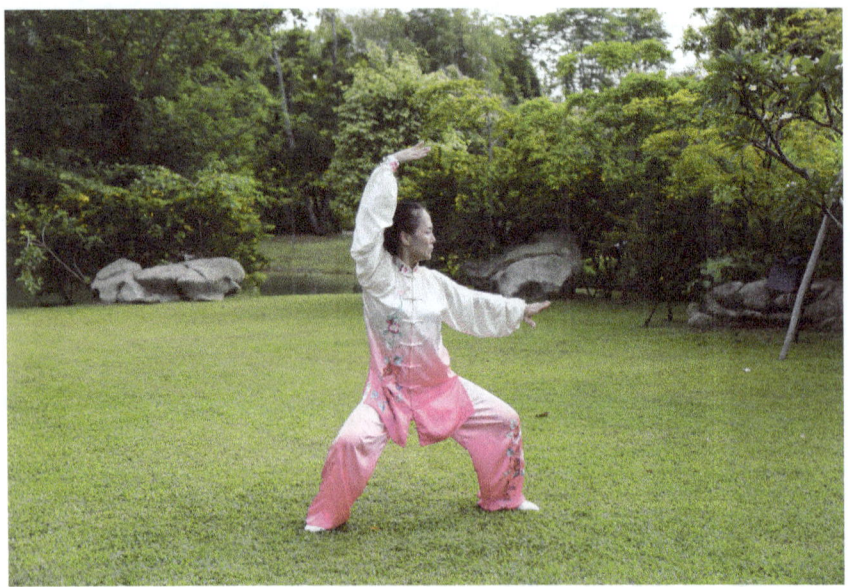

Fig. 6.141.

The left leg pushes off, and the body's center of gravity moves quickly between the front legs or a bit more to the right leg, while the right arm and palm is raised quickly, with the right elbow slightly bent, and the right arm staying bent. The right palm faces toward the lower left, stopping above the head. The left palm bumps forward, and the left arm stays straight naturally, at a height of about chest level. Look in the direction of the left palm (east) (Fig. 6.141).

48. Right wiping palm

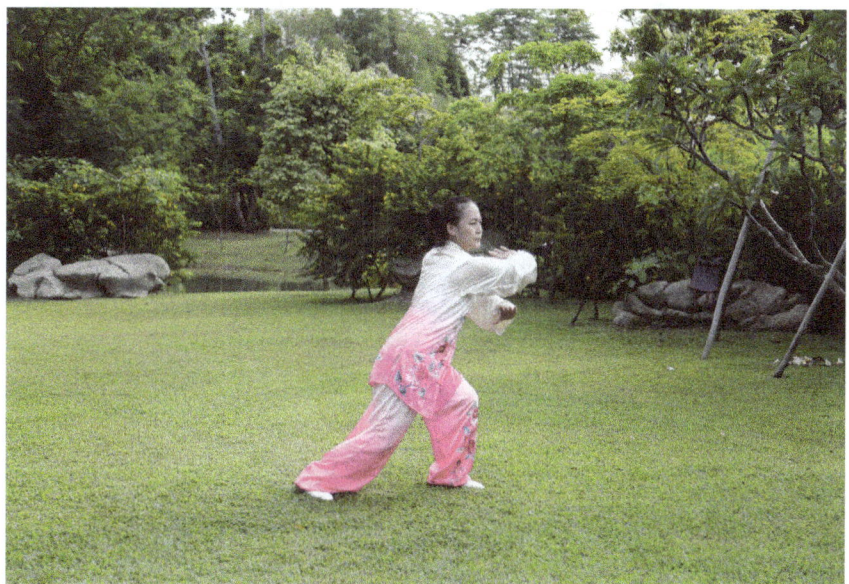

Fig. 6.142.

1. Move the center of gravity of the body slightly to the left and turn left. While the left arm is bending, the left palm begins to swing to the right and then to the back in an arc. The right palm moves lower down to the lower left above the left arm (Fig. 6.142).

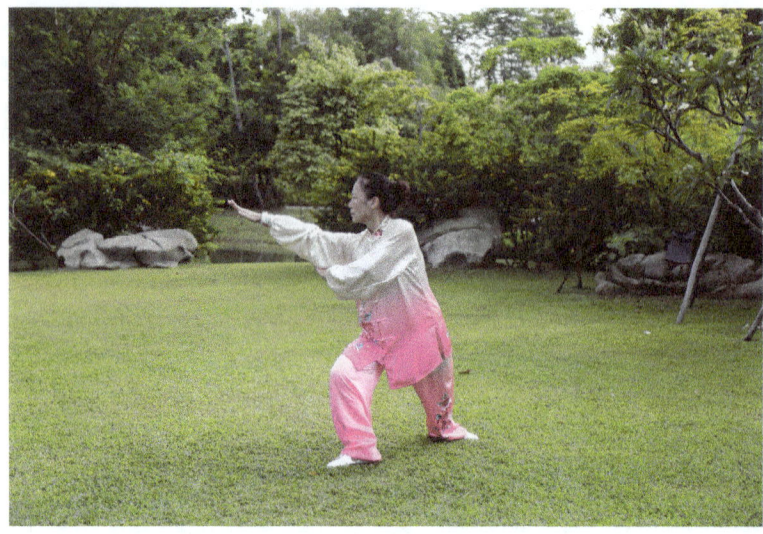

Fig. 6.143.

2. Turn right, and to move the center of gravity of the body toward the right leg, the right foot can adjust the step naturally. At the same time, the right arm extends straight, while the right palm wipes horizontally toward the right, then the back (west), in a wide range. The left palm swings rightward along and under the right arm to the right chest, both palms facing down. Look toward the right palm (Fig. 6.143).

49. Left wiping palm

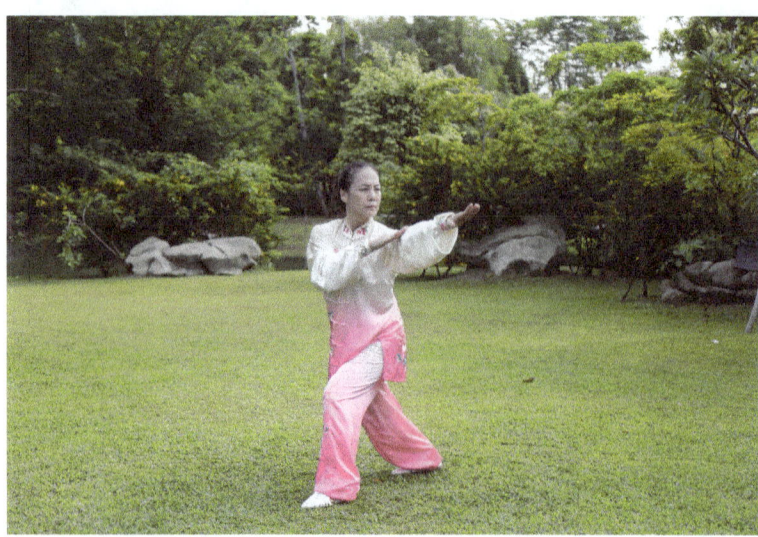

Fig. 6.144.

The left foot steps forward to the southwest, and the left palm wipes horizontally toward the front, then left, in a wide range. The right palm swings toward the left and then the back to the left chest, both palms facing down. Look toward the left palm (Fig. 6.144).

Key Points

The two wiping palms should be performed continuously without stopping. The strides should be wide and swift without making a sound while landing. Stay low in the process.

50. Right tuck-in palm

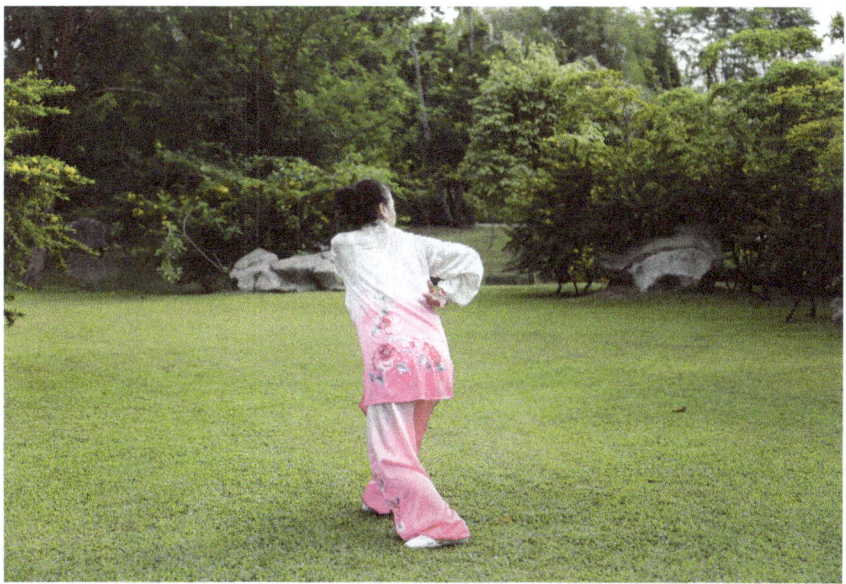

Fig. 6.145.

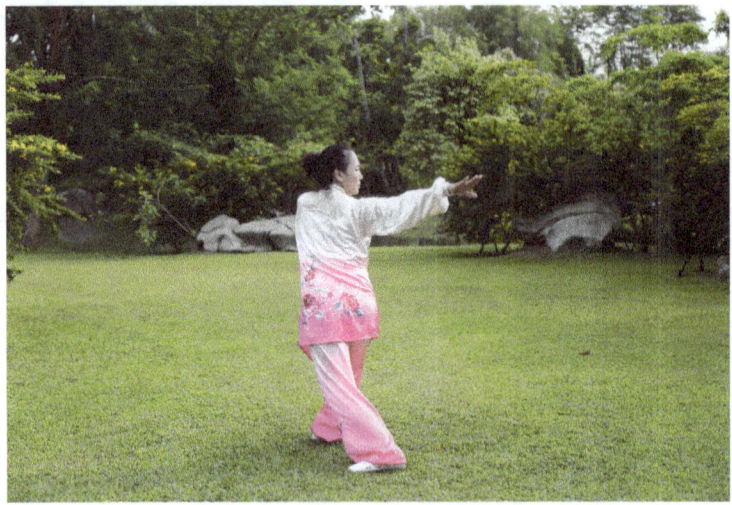

Fig. 6.146.

The body turns right into the position facing north. Move the center of gravity of the body toward the right leg, and the right foot can adjust the step naturally. At the same time, the right palm turns anti-clockwise to face up, and then turns inward with the right wrist bent near the right ribs, and thrust out toward the right back. The left arm bends, and the left hand swings toward the right and then the back to reach the right armpit. Look toward the right palm (Figs. 6.145 and 6.146).

51. Left wiping palm

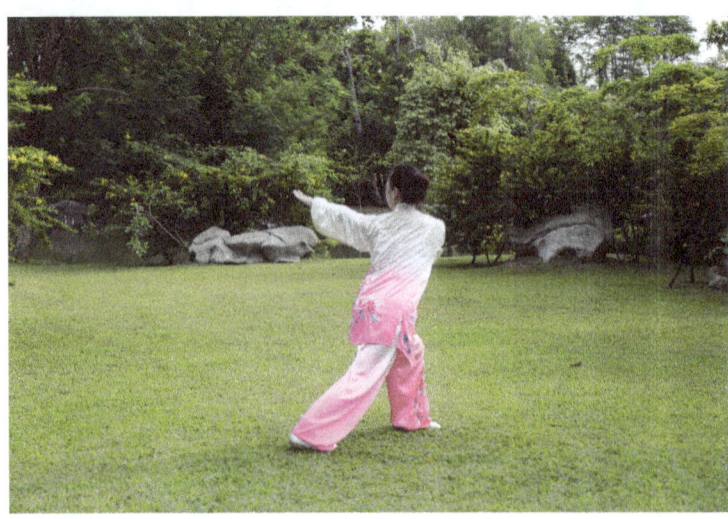

Fig. 6.147.

The left foot steps forward to perform the inward-latching step to the southwest. At the same time, the left palm wipes horizontally toward the front and left in a wide arc. The right palm swings toward the left and then the back to reach the left shoulder. Look toward the left palm (Fig. 6.147).

52. Right wiping palm

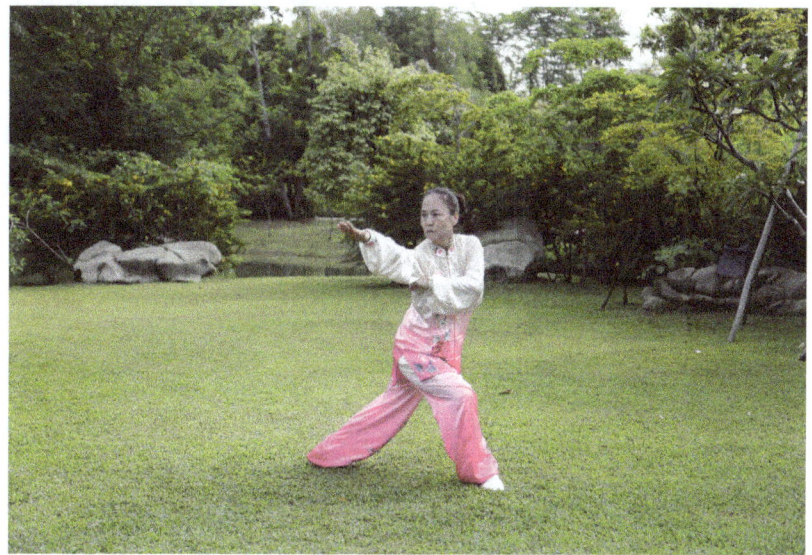

Fig. 6.148.

The body turns right, and the right foot steps forward to perform the outward-swinging step to the northeast. At the same time, the right palm wipes horizontally toward the left front, then right in a wide arc. The left palm swings toward the right and then the back to the right chest. Look toward the right palm (Fig. 6.148).

Key Points

1. The change of the angles of the steps and the range of the arm swing and body turning should be tuned to personal situations rather than be fixed.
2. The head turning should be performed with flashing eyes and present an air of being capable of covering both sides with a sense of elusiveness in terms of which direction to attack.
3. All the wiping palms should be performed with the palms facing down.

53. Left tuck-in palm

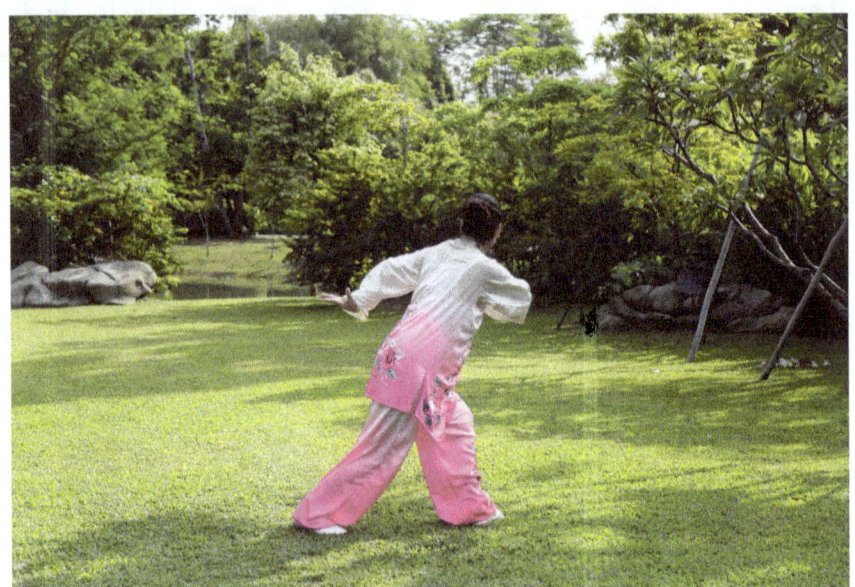

Fig. 6.149.

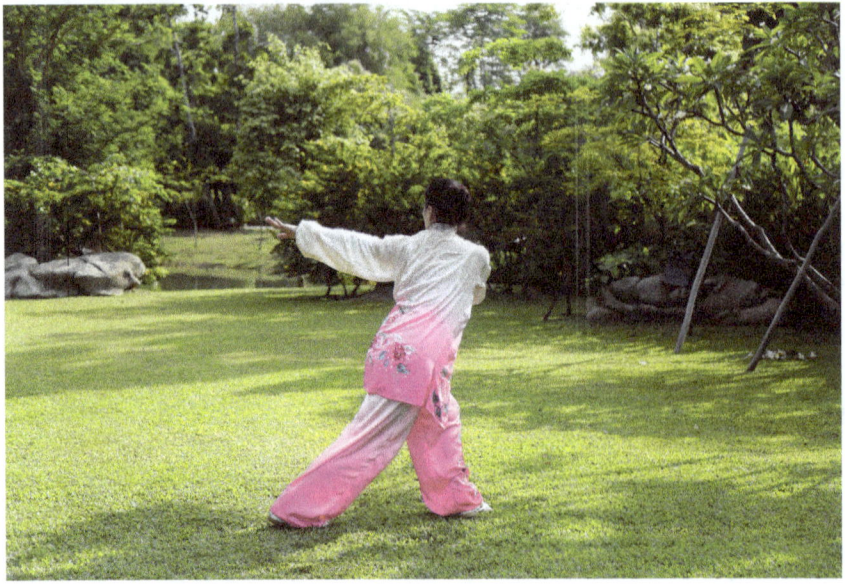

Fig. 6.150.

The body turns left, and the left palm tucks in near the left ribs and thrusts out toward the left. At the same time, the right palm withdraws to reach the chest. Look toward the left palm (Figs. 6.149 and 6.150).

54. Joint holding palms

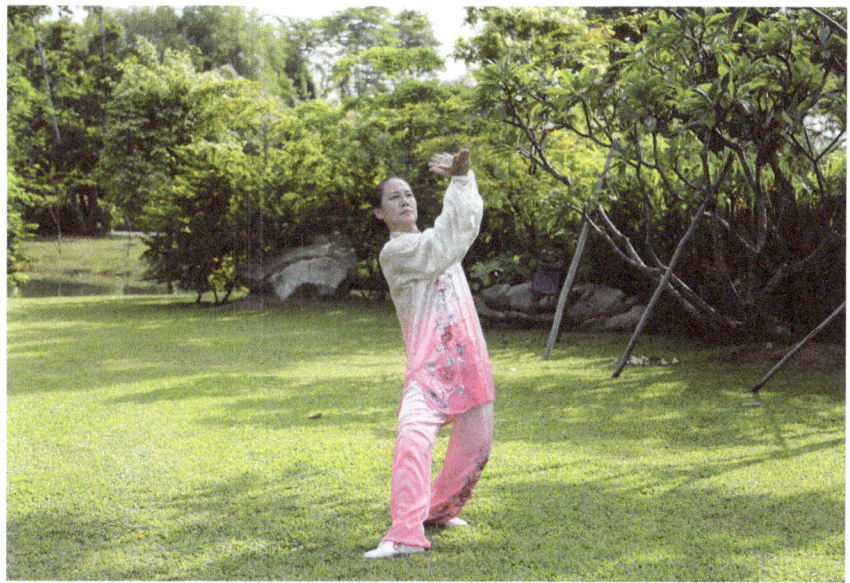

Fig. 6.151.

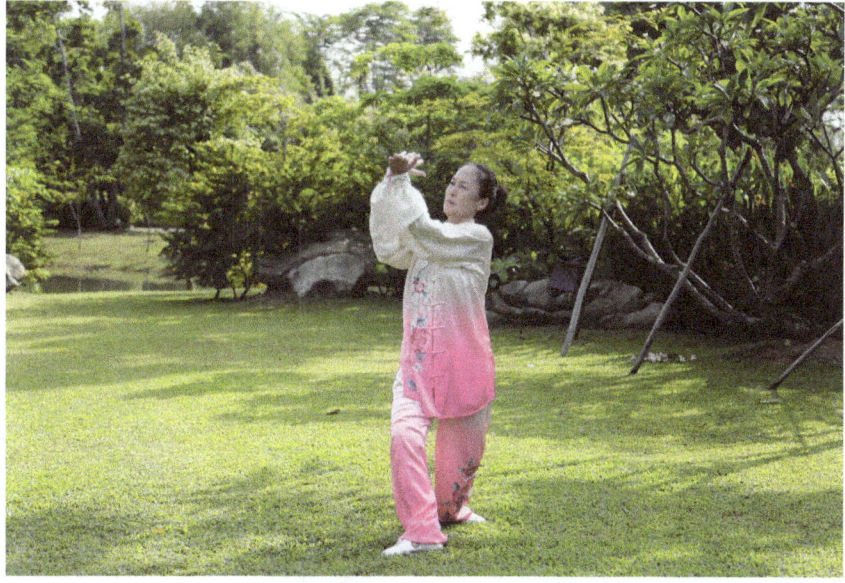

Fig. 6.152.

The right foot moves forward to perform an outward swing step to the right and then the front (south) in an arc, and the body turns right. The palms should naturally be raised above the head in front, palms touching each other at the base. Rotate with the body to the right, head slightly leaning back, looking at the palms (Figs. 6.151 and 6.152).

55. Turn with drilling palms

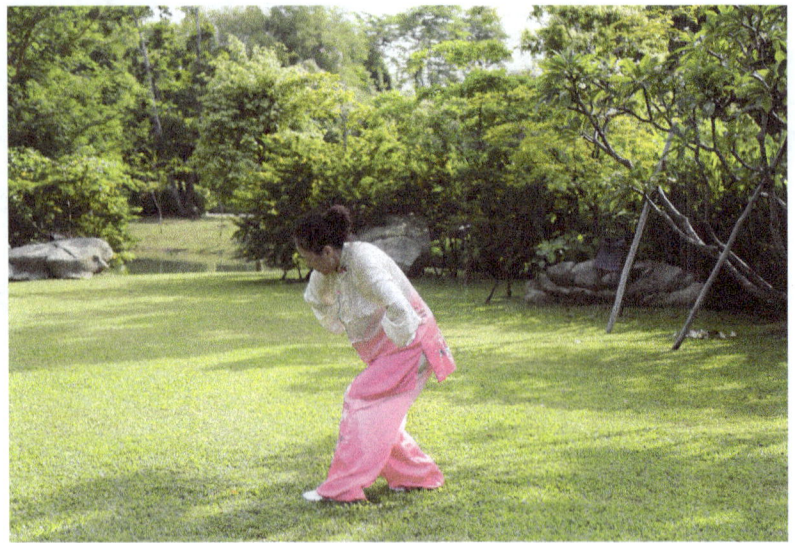

Fig. 6.153.

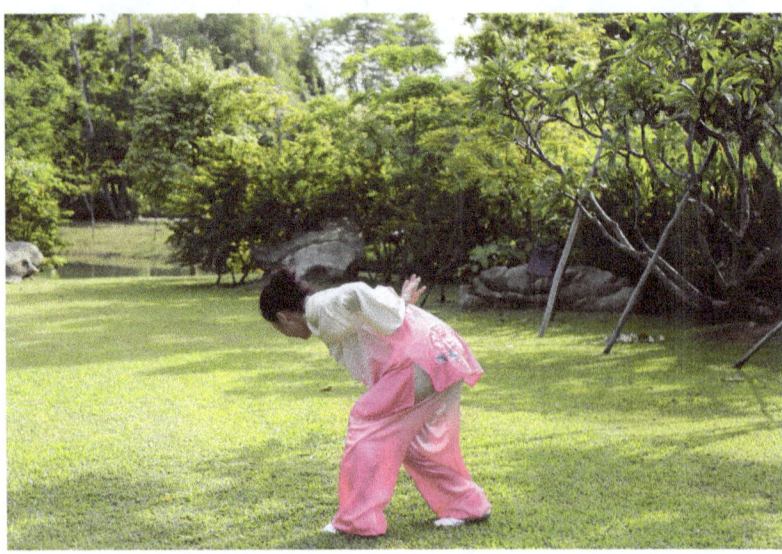

Fig. 6.154.

1. Step the left foot southwest to perform the inward-latching step. The body continues to turn right, with the upper body leaning forward and lowering gradually in the process. Meanwhile, the palms rotate to the extreme right, then roll into the position where the back of the palms touch each other. Next, immediately bend the wrists and move downward, and then backward to insert to the sides of the flanks, with the fingertips pointing toward the upper back side. The head turns right (Fig. 6.153 and 6.154).

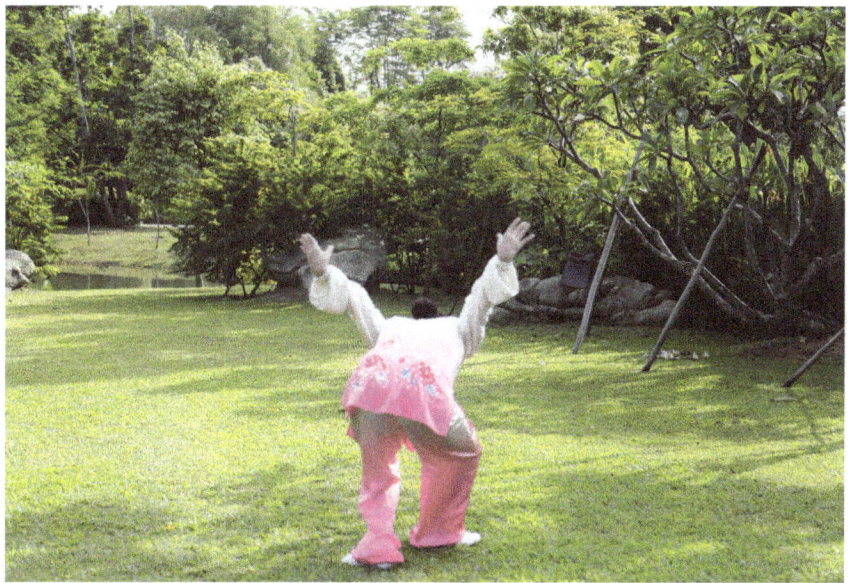

Fig. 6.155.

2. The body continues to turn right, stepping the right foot toward the northeast to perform the outward swing. The palms continue to drill toward the upper back side, with the arms straight, and fingers pointed upward (Fig. 6.155).

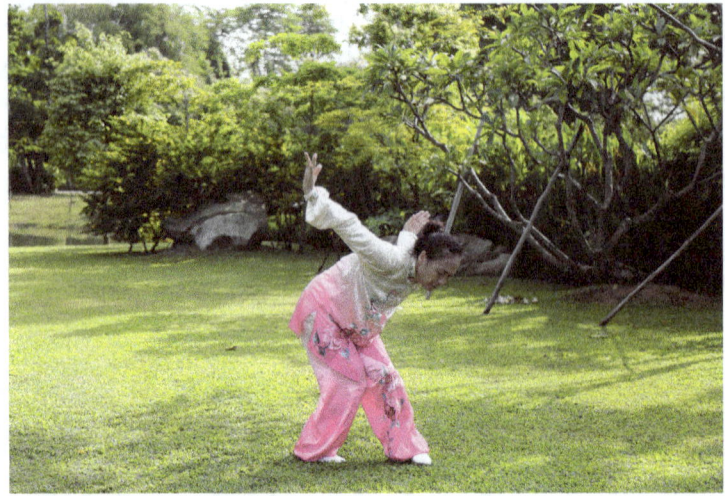

Fig. 6.156.

3. The body continues to turn right, and the left foot steps eastward to perform the inward-latching step, while the arms turn right with the body (Fig. 6.156).

Key Points

In practice, this form can be performed with sudden acceleration, and the body should stay low.

56. Holding up palms

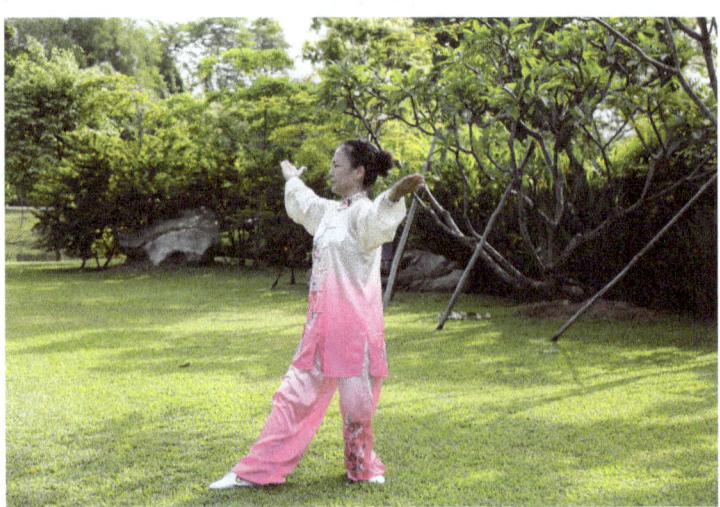

Fig. 6.157.

The right foot performs the outward-swinging step to the right, then the mud-wading steps with the upper body kept upright. Both hands turn to have palms facing up and holding up, with the arms naturally straight, and the palms slightly higher than the shoulders (Fig. 6.157).

57. Joint holding palms

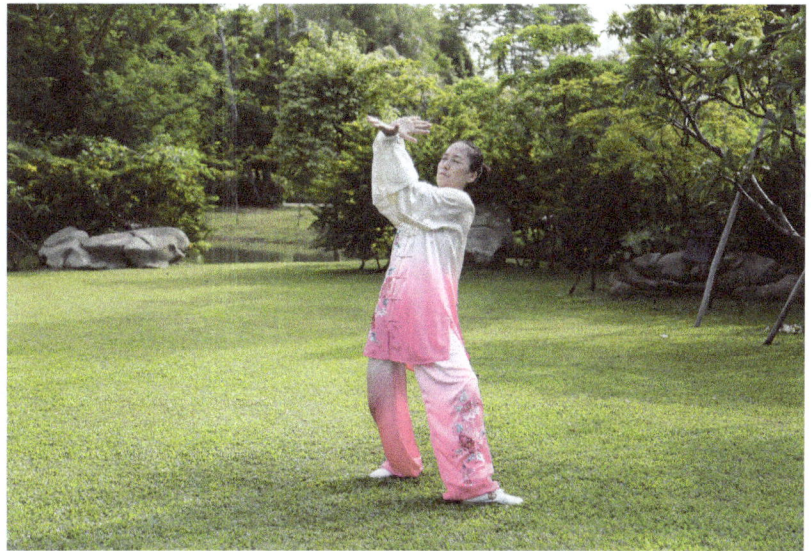

Fig. 6.158.

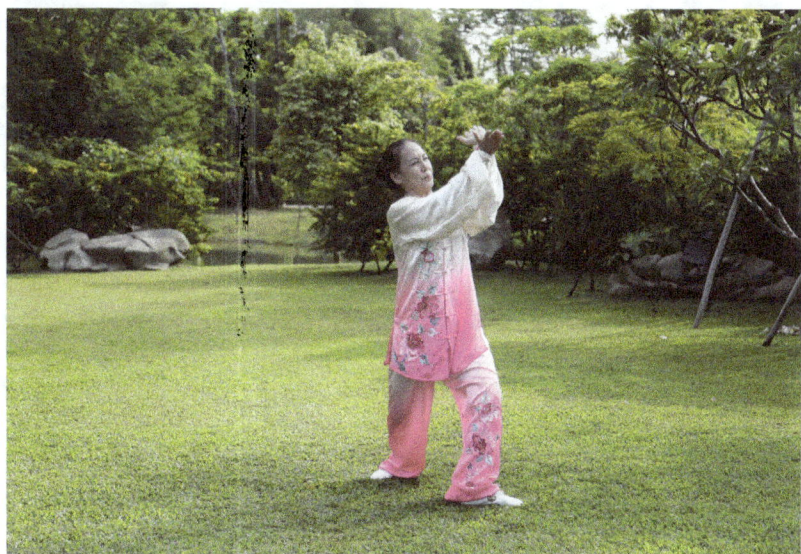

Fig. 6.159.

After two steps toward the right in an arc in the previous form, turn left abruptly and perform an outward-swinging step. At the same time, with the left turning of the body, the palms rise in front and above the head with crossing and twisting. Firstly, arms quickly move close to each other and twist inward. When the wrists cross over, the right palm is closer to the body, with the palm facing the front right, tilted; the left palm is placed outside the right palm, palm facing the front left, tilted. Then the palms touch at the base and rotate to form a cup, then continue to turn to the left with the body. The head slightly leans back (Figs. 6.158 and 6.159).

Key Points

This form can also be performed starting from the inward-latching step of the right foot and then rotating to the left. The practitioner can decide based on personal habits. If you select to start from the inward-latching step of the right foot, then you may start to perform the inward-latching step immediately after one or three steps.

58. Left heaven drilling palm

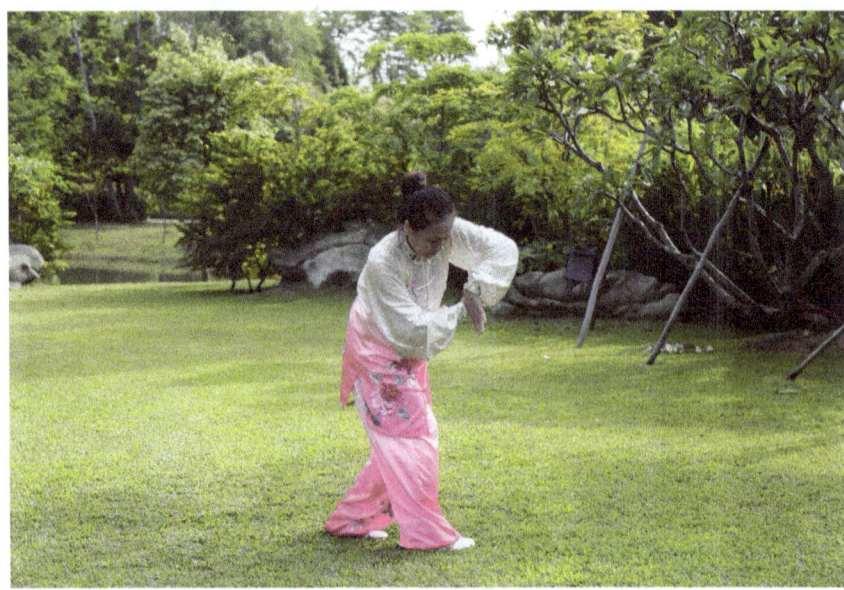

Fig. 6.160.

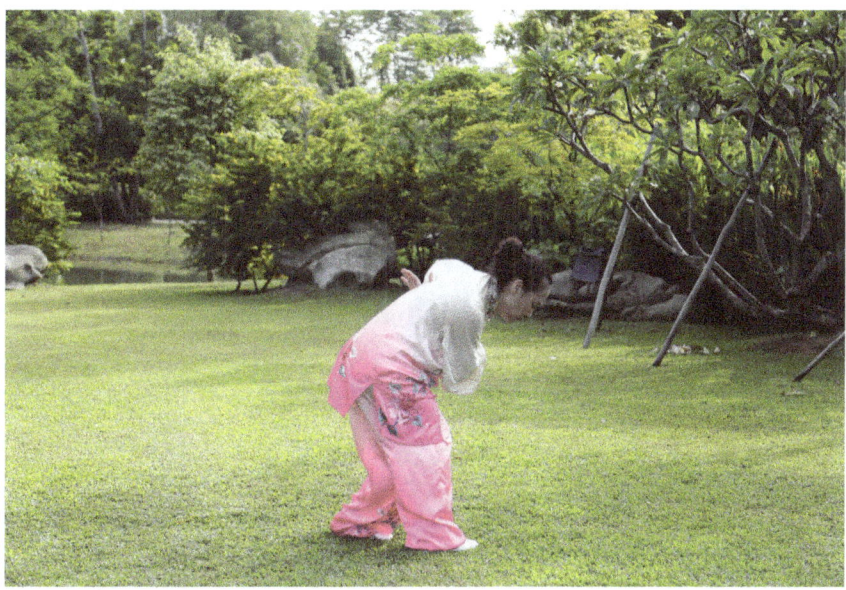

Fig. 6.161.

1. The right foot moves over the left foot with an inward-latching step. The palms continue to rotate downward, while the left palm closes in with wrist bending inward to thrust toward the side of the left rib (Figs. 6.160 and 6.161).

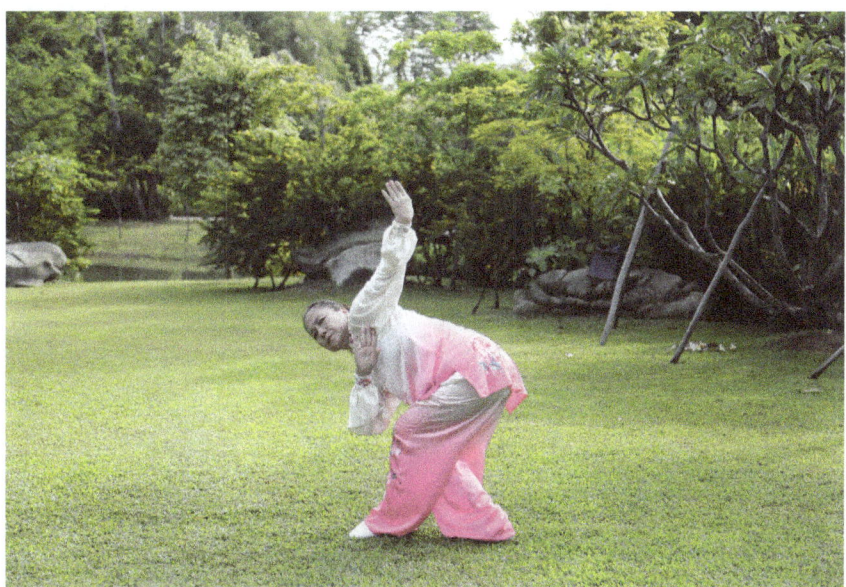

Fig. 6.162.

2. The left foot swings outward, while the left palm continues to drill toward the upper back side from the side of the left rib, and the left arm stretches straight. At the same time, the upper body leans forward more, the head turns to the extreme left, and the right palm stays in front of the left chest (Fig. 6.162).

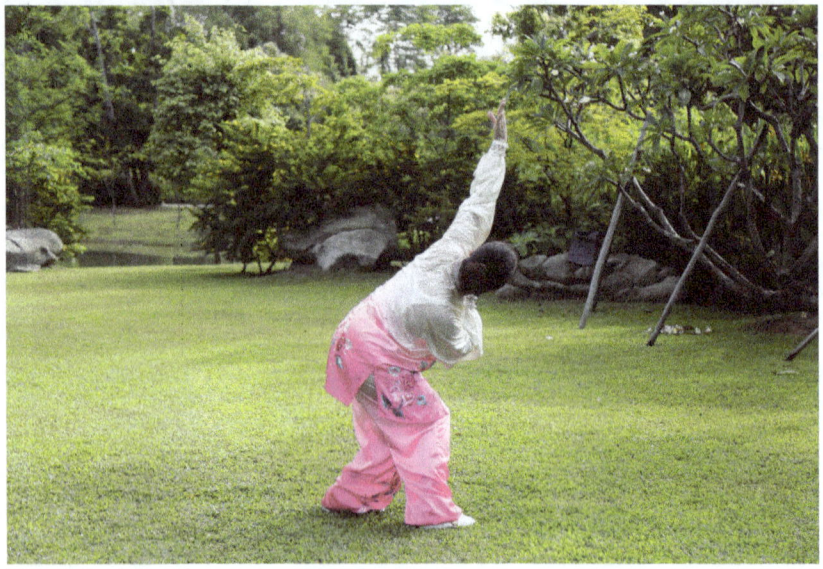

Fig. 6.163.

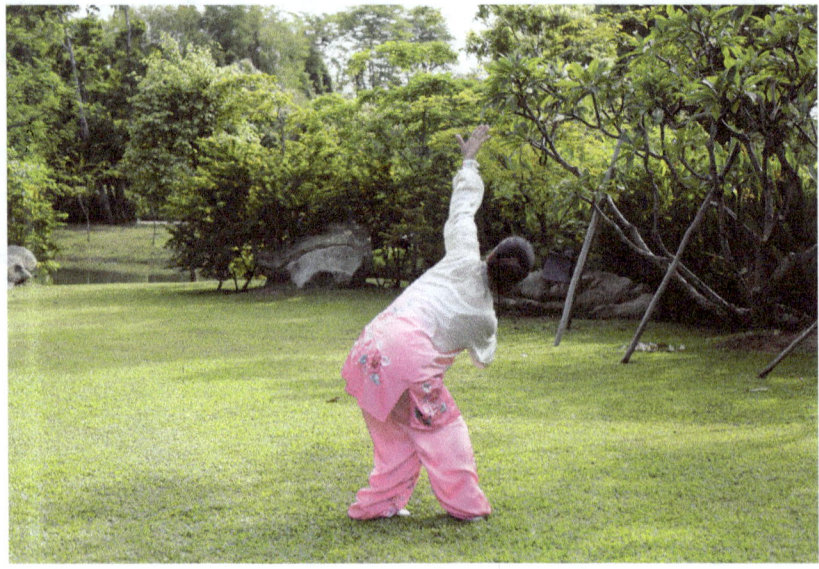

Fig. 6.164.

3. The right foot performs an inward-latching step, and the left foot swings outward. Continue these footwork combinations. The upper body maintains the same position relative to the palms and rotates toward the left with the stepping foot while the speed accelerates. The number of steps is decided by personal preference, and the route should be small and circular. The upper body should be raised gradually at the end (Figs. 6.163 and 6.164).

Key Points

1. The steps of this form should be small and fast.
2. The body weight is always a little closer to the left, which is closer to the center of the circle, so it is easier to go with the inertia, which makes the move smooth and easier to speed up naturally.

59. Horizontal pushing palm

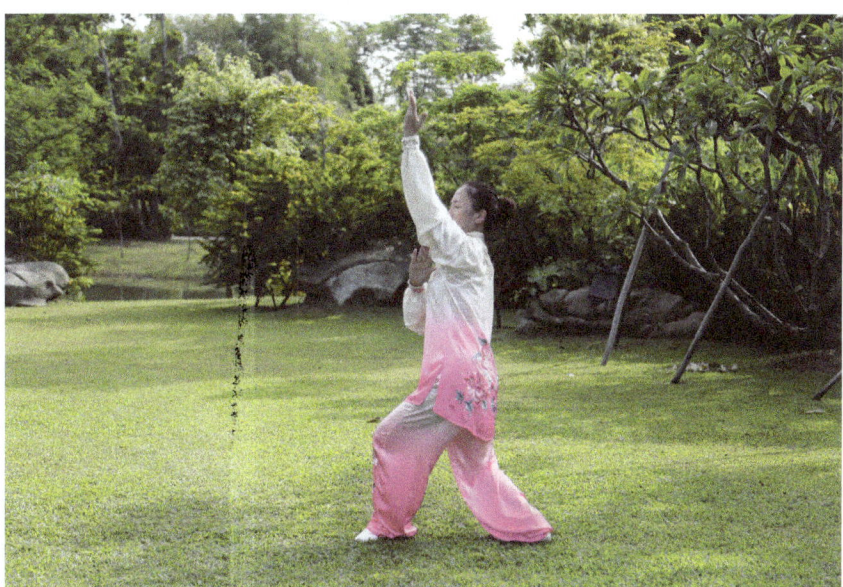

Fig. 6.165.

1. When facing west with the rotating of the previous form, the upper body will be almost upright (Fig. 6.165).

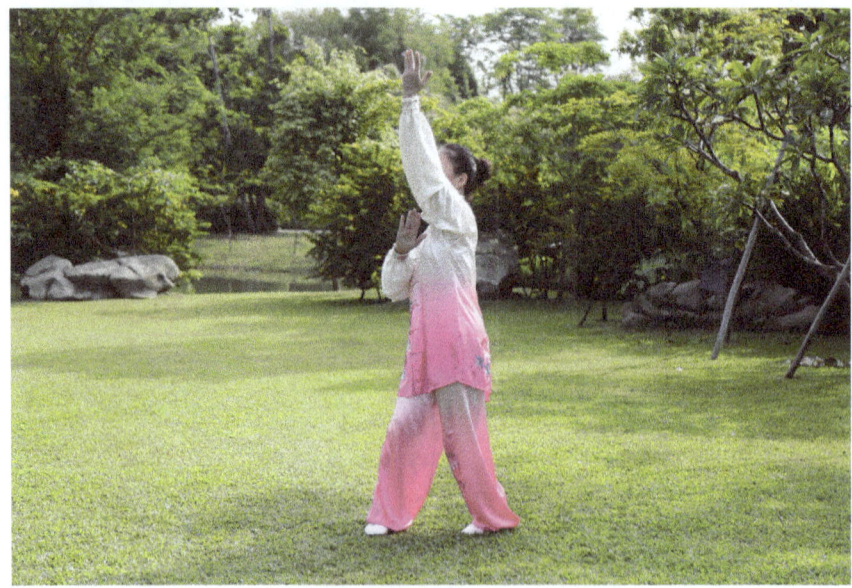

Fig. 6.166.

Next, the right foot performs an inward-latching step to the west (Fig. 6.166).

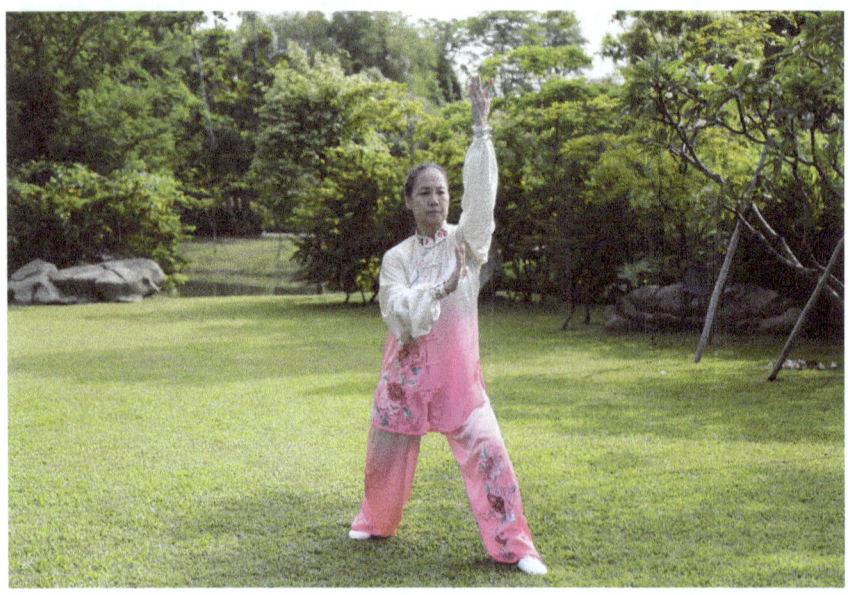

Fig. 6.167.

2. The left foot strides to the east for half a step (Fig. 6.167).

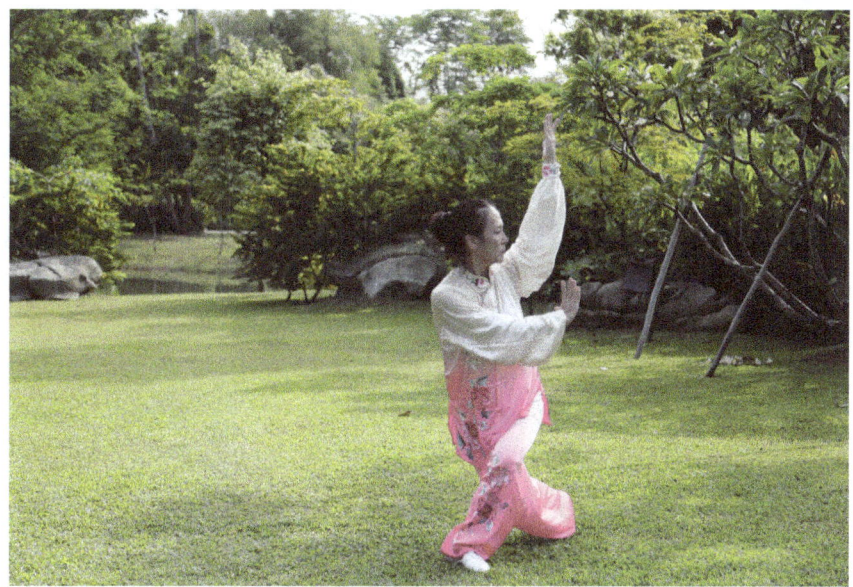

Fig. 6.168.

With the momentum of the last move toward the east, the right foot steps rapidly eastward from behind the left leg to form a back cross-step. The ball of the foot touches the ground, and the body weight stays on the right side. While the right palm pushes from the chest to the left horizontally, the left hand stays raised, pointing up to the sky. Look toward the direction of the pushing palm (Fig. 6.168).

Key Points

Stay low while performing the back cross-step, with the body weight staying on the right side to prepare properly for the instant rightward opening stance in the next form.

60. Open stance up pushing palm

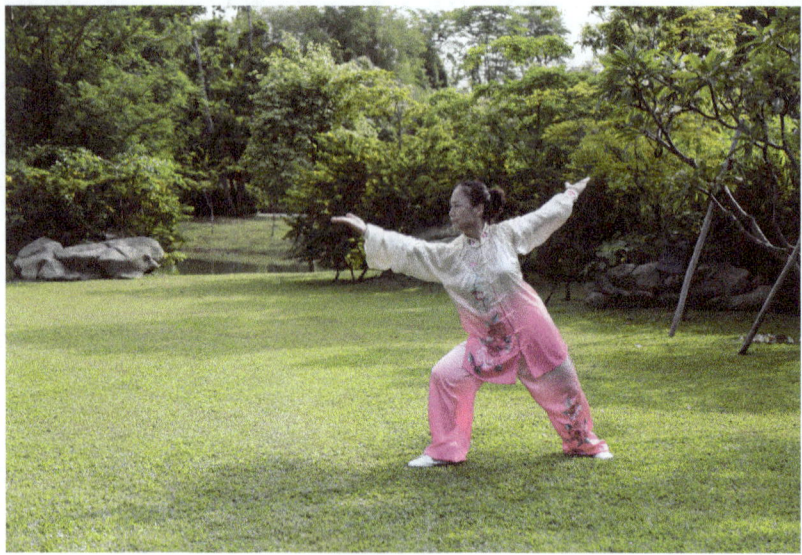

Fig. 6.169.

1. Continuing from the previous form, the right foot strides immediately westward. At the same time, the right palm quickly swings to the front, and then to the right in an arc, palms facing up. Drop the left arm and turn the head right (Fig. 6.169).

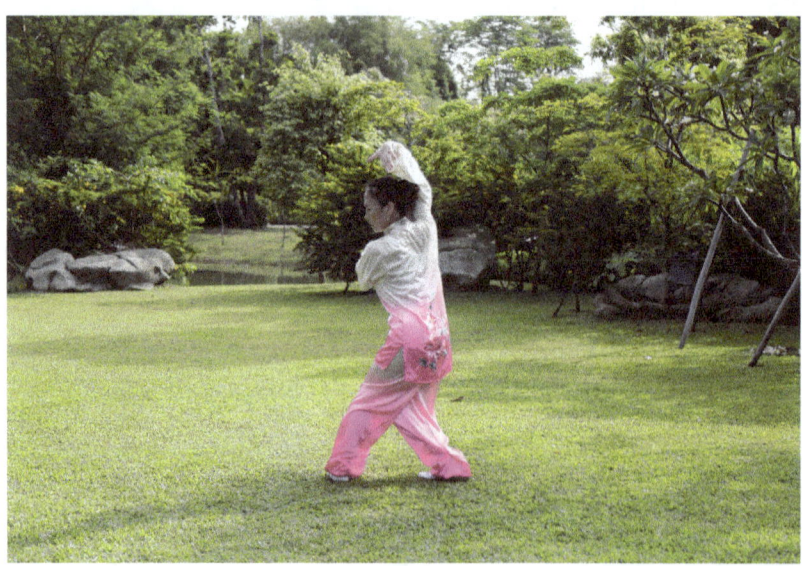

Fig. 6.170.

2. Move the left foot westward to form an inward-latching step. The body turns right, the right arm bends, and the right palm swings to the rear until reaching behind the upper right shoulder and then pushes up, palm facing up and the fingers pointing left, the right elbow slightly bent. At the same time, turn right while the left palm swings rightward with the body, then bend to swing the left palm to reach under the right armpit, palm facing toward the lower right (Fig. 6.170).

61. Hugging palm with folded body

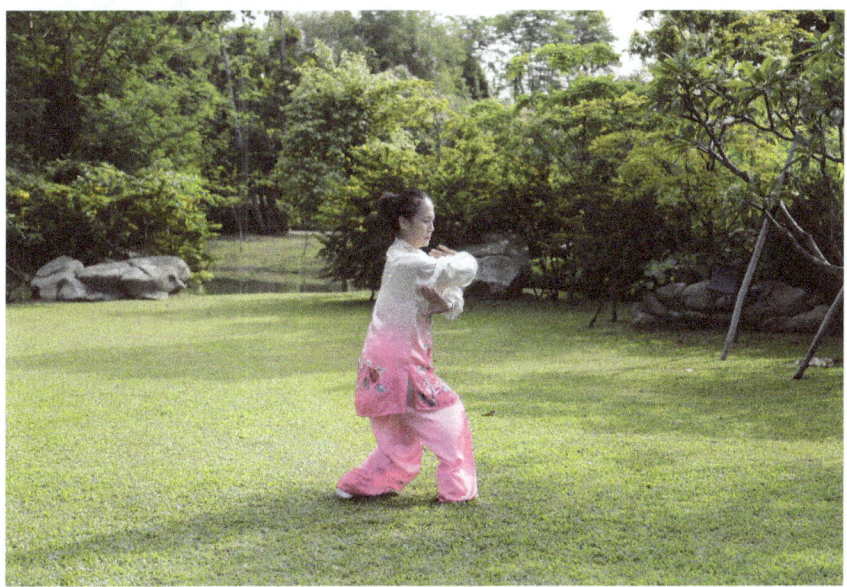

Fig. 6.171.

The body continues to turn right. The right palm continues to perform cloud palm and then falls beside the left shoulder, palm facing the lower left. The left palm remains under the right armpit, with the arms held together in a circle with a folded body, right arm on top (Fig. 6.171).

62. Double-pressing palm after a turn

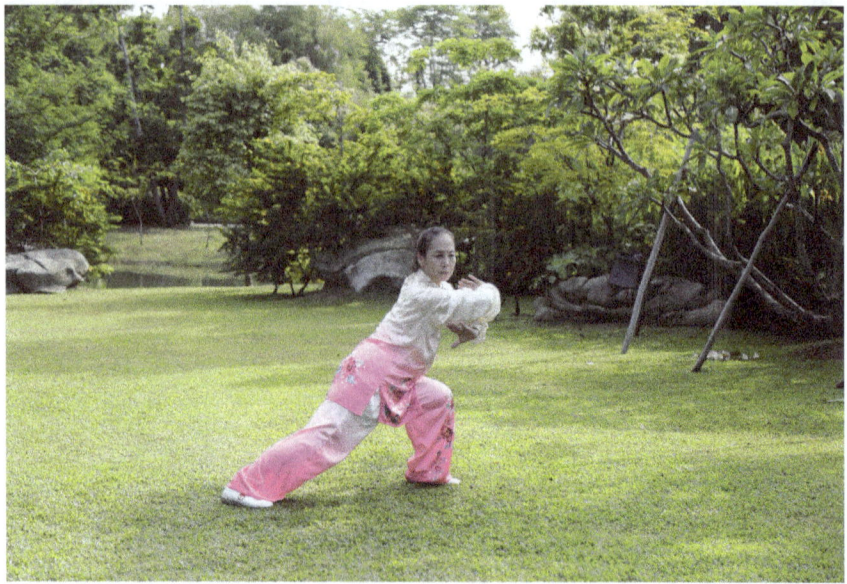

Fig. 6.172.

The right foot rapidly steps backward to the west, and the body continues to turn right (Fig. 6.172).

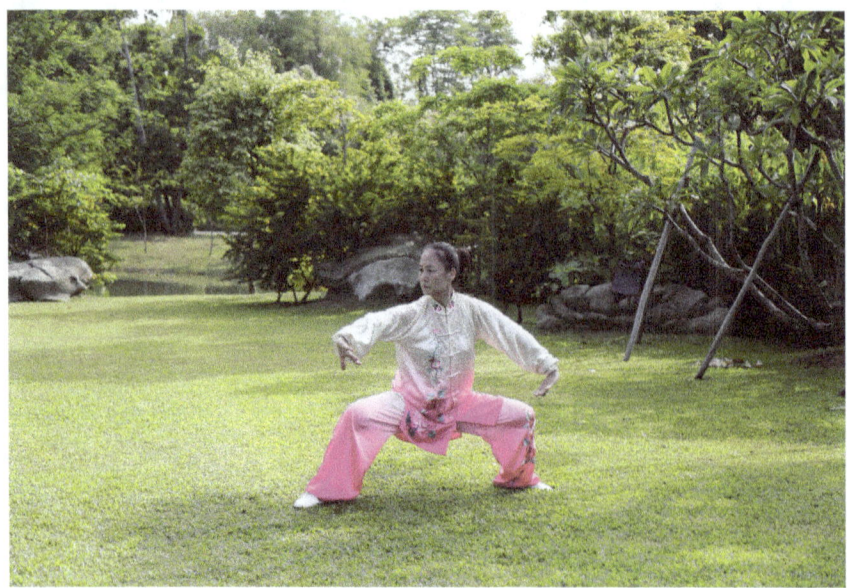

Fig. 6.173.

Next, the body's center of gravity moves to the right between the legs. Squat with the knees bent, keeping the upper body straight (Fig. 6.173).

At the same time, with the momentum of the rightward shift of the body, the palms press down, tilted from the left and right side. The thumbs and index fingers separate wide apart to form a convex pointing to the body or slightly toward the front. The arms form an arc. Look toward the right palm (Fig. 6.173).

63. Right piercing palm with inward-latching step

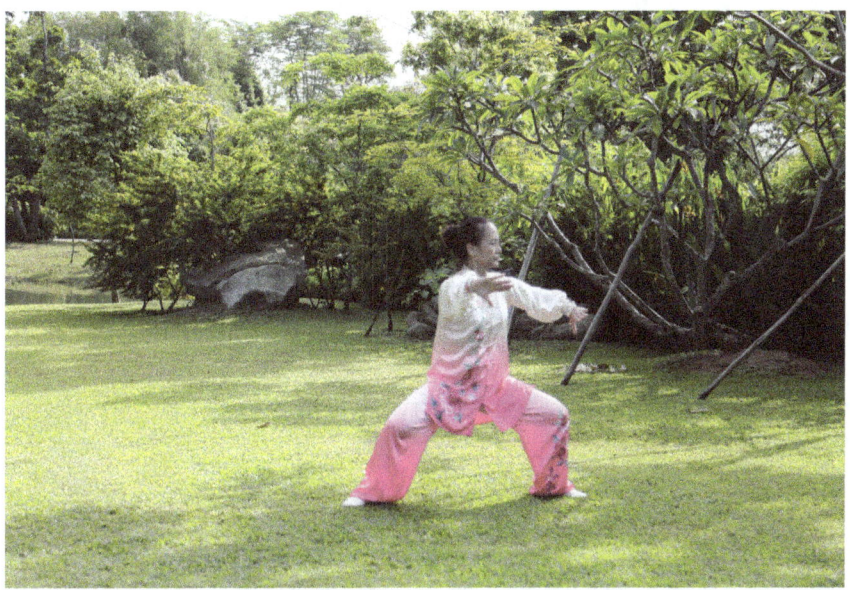

Fig. 6.174.

1. The body turns slightly to the left, and the head turns left with it. The arms naturally swing to the upper left with this momentum, staying slightly bent and arched. The right palm stays at about the same height as the shoulder, with the left palm lower than the shoulders, and the head turned left (Fig. 6.174).

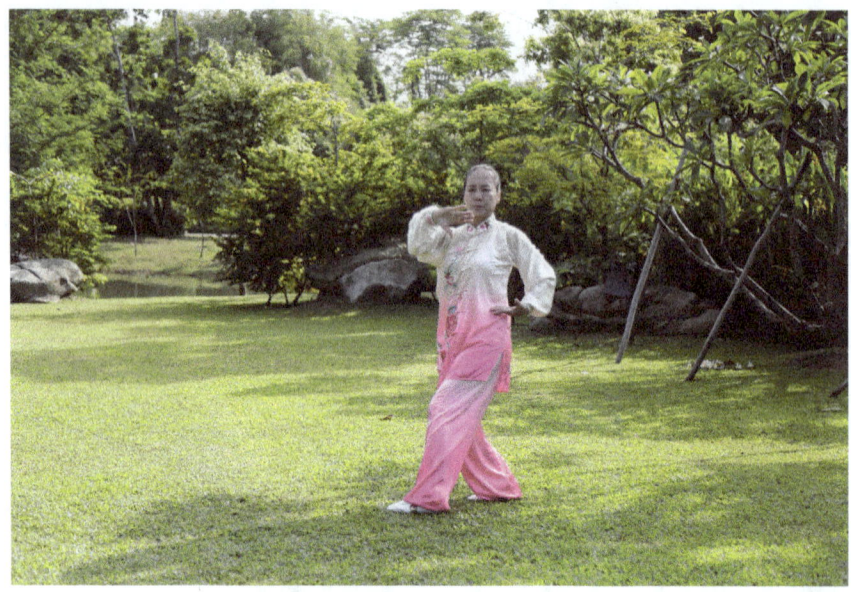

Fig. 6.175.

2. The body quickly turns right, and the head also turns right with it. The left foot moves forward rapidly to perform the inward-latching step in front of the right toes. The right palm swings to the right in an arc with the momentum, and the left palm rotates anti-clockwise and stays close to the left waist, palm facing up (Fig. 6.175).

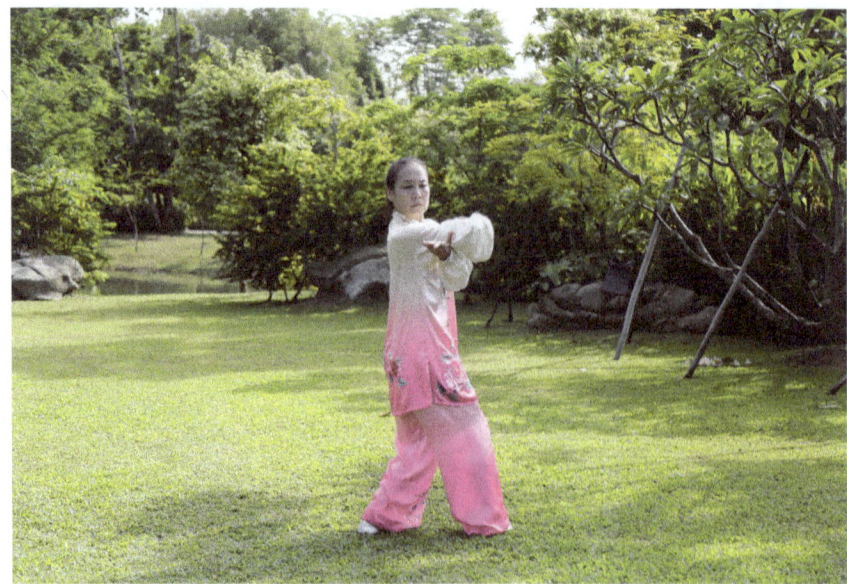

Fig. 6.176.

3. The body and the head continue to turn right, and the left palm pierces out along the chest to the right armpit. At the same time, the right arm bends, and the right palm touches the outside of the left shoulder, palm facing outward. Look to the right (Fig. 6.176).

64. Left push palm

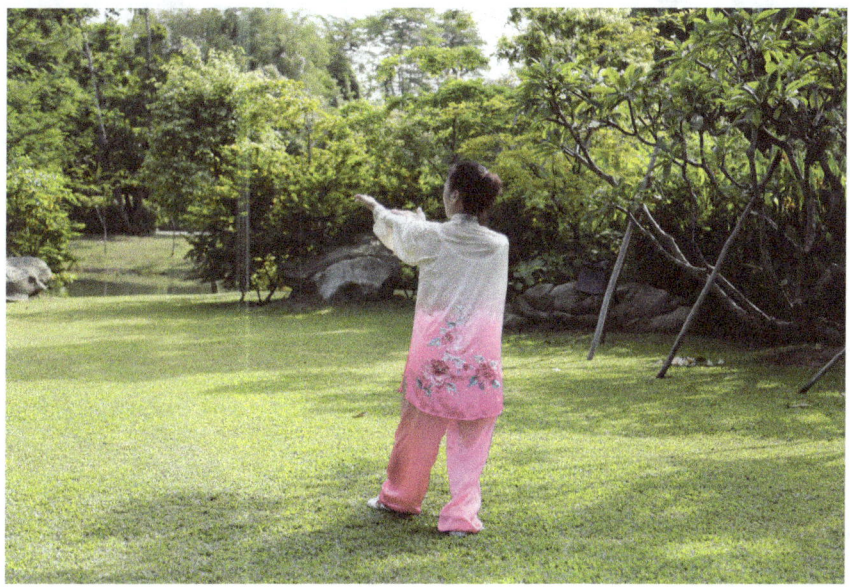

Fig. 6.177.

1. The body turns left, and the left palm pierces out along the outer lower side of the right arm, going forward and outside, and then leftward, in an arc. At the same time, the right palm moves away from the left shoulder and extends forward, rotating clockwise to face up. As the left palm is extending forward, the right palm pulls back to be placed on top of the left arm. Step forward with the left foot to the northwest with an outward swing, looking toward the left palm (Fig. 6.177).

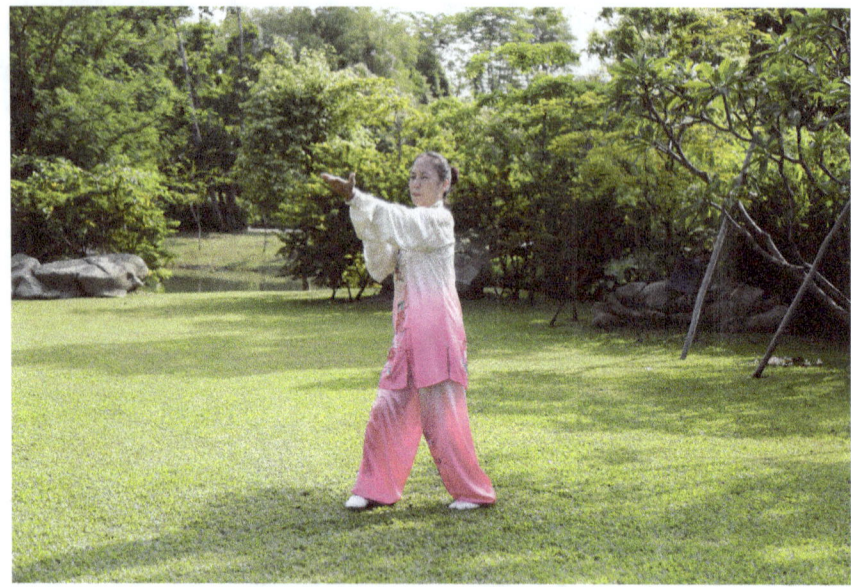

Fig. 6.178.

2. Without stopping from the last move, the right foot performs an inward-latching step to the west. The body keeps turning left, and the palms start to swing to the left. Rotate the arms inward — the left palm turns clockwise and the right palm turns anti-clockwise (Fig. 6.178).

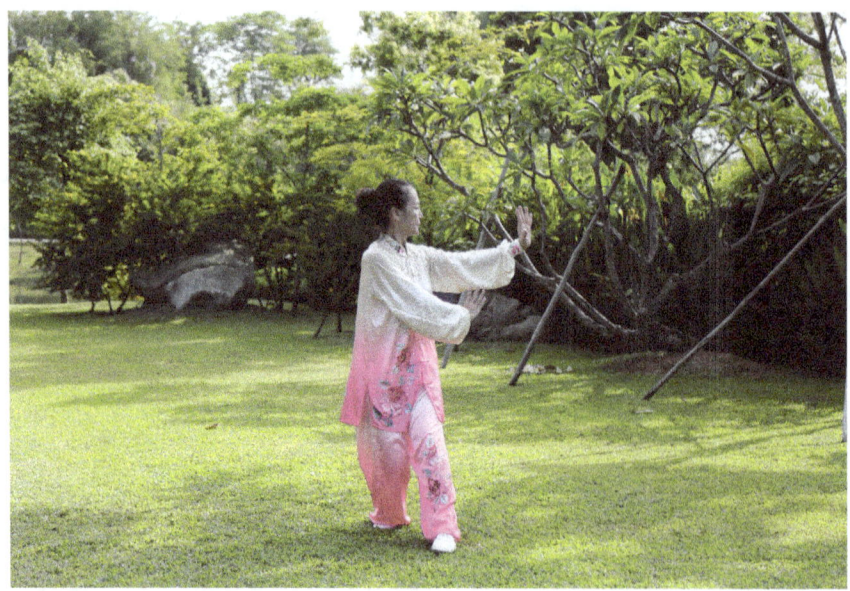

Fig. 6.179.

3. The left foot wades forward toward the south, the upper body continues to turn left, and the arms and palms continue to swing leftward to the back, the wrists extruding out with the fingers turned up. The right palm drops toward the underside of the left elbow, and the upper body twists to the left as much as possible. Look toward the left palm. The requirements for the palms are the same as in form 2, step 4 (Fig. 6.179).

Key Points

1. Feel free to change the number of steps. The key is to go back to roughly the same place and direction as the initial form.
2. As for the rhythm of the performance:
    (1) If there are many steps, move at the same speed and stop gradually.
    (2) If there are only two steps, go fast and reduce the speed later to showcase the power.

Closing form

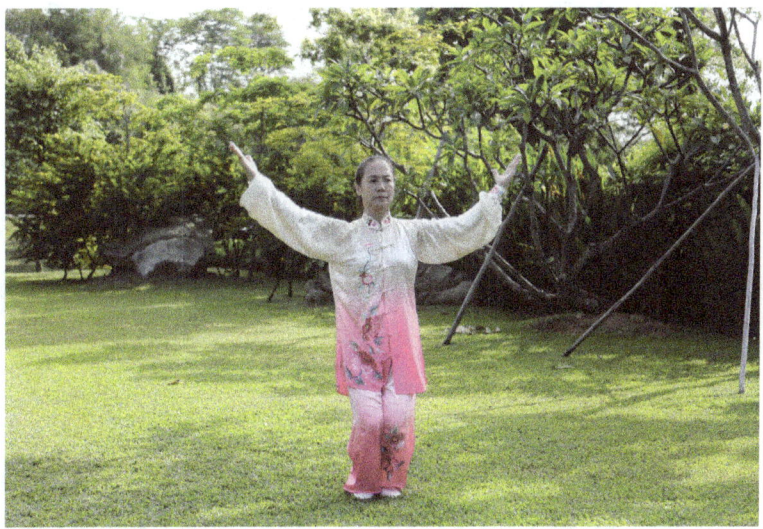

Fig. 6.180.

1. Move the body weight forward. The right foot steps forward to come close with the left foot. The knees stay close while the legs bend, and the upper body stays straight and relaxed. At the same time, the right palm swings to the right and then upward. The palms rotate to face up, stretching the arms to the sides with palms higher than the shoulders (Fig. 6.180).

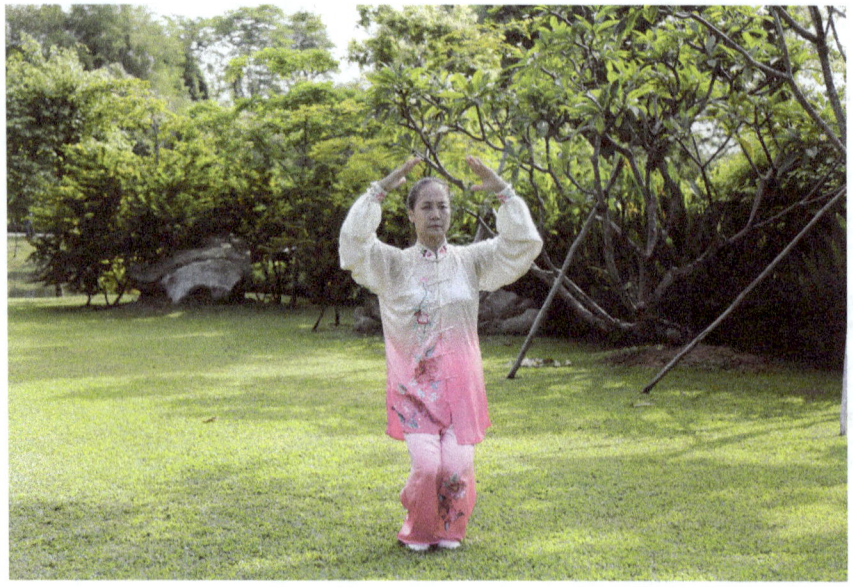

Fig. 6.181.

2. Fold the arms, with the hands coming close to each other with the wrists bent, the fingers of the hands pointing to each other tilted, and the palms facing downward tilted (Fig. 6.181).

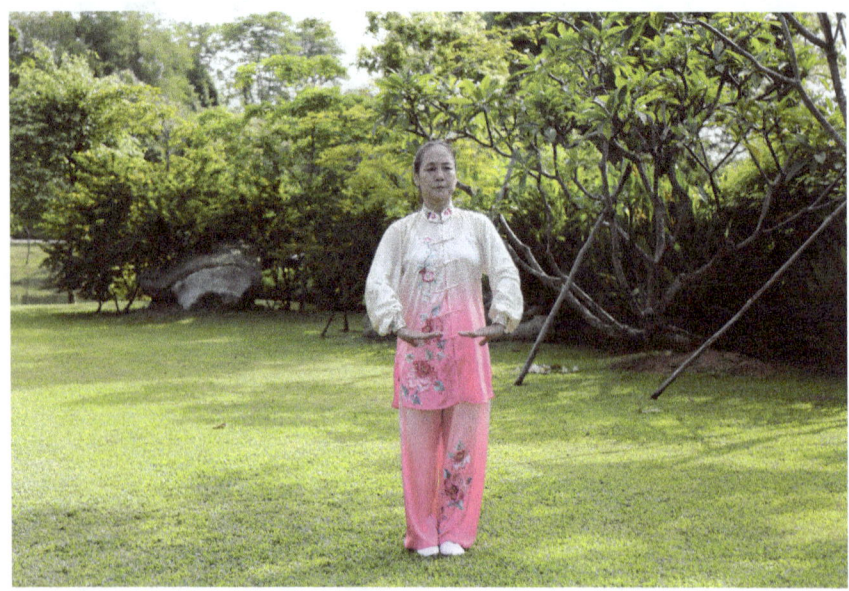

Fig. 6.182.

3. Push off with the legs and stand up gradually. Push down the palms gradually until reaching the front of the abdomen. Keep the palms facing down and the arms slightly bent (Fig. 6.182).

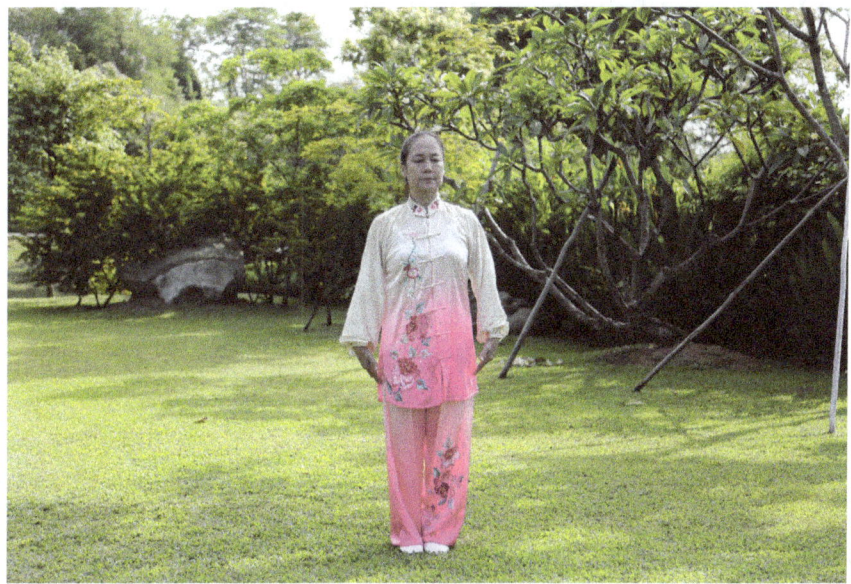

Fig. 6.183.

Finally, relax the elbows and wrists, letting the arms hang loose beside the body. The closing form is done (Fig. 6.183).

Appendix I: Key Notes on Martial Art Training

1. In essence, no matter what the training or performance of the forms may be, the martial arts are all about the stance and movement of the body, and the rhythm and style of the whole set. So the trainer and trainee should study the key rules and specialties of each form as well as the basic style of the martial arts. Train in scientific ways after understanding the basics of the style and try your best to realize it in actual performance. The most difficult part is actually the stance, taste, and style of the martial art. So it is not advisable to train blindly, but to study with a humble mind and scrutinize everything to finally realize the secrets of the art.
2. To achieve the requirements above, slower exercises should be applied to gain the feeling about the correct route and delicate stance changes, inner feelings, and so on. Trainees should not just remember with their heart but with their muscles, so that whenever a movement is not up to standard, they will feel it and correct it. When a pattern is formed for certain movements, they can speed up gradually and finally train at normal speed.
3. To handle the relationship between exercises of the separated parts of the forms, single forms, grouped forms, form period, and the whole form properly, assign the right formula of proportions and cycles. Strengthen the single form practice and even the exercises of the separated parts of the forms, before proceeding to the group forms. This method will allow trainees to focus better with a clearer mind and enough energy to follow the requirements properly to ensure quality training. It also helps them to remember the movements properly. Try to get trainees to eliminate repeating errors during training, or these will go into their memory and become hard to fix.
4. The martial art team should set priorities for different types of training at different periods, following the set schedules of competitions. The rigor of the training should firstly be built on the basis of a set of strictly defined specifications of each movement. Any training should target a very specific purpose without blindly repeating anything. The trainees need to understand what problems need to be solved and where the target is, and train accordingly. This will enable them to train with interest and purpose so that each time they train, they will be able to

identify the problem and know where they have reached the target and where they need more improvements. This will not only keep the trainees' spirits high but also ensure the high quality of the training and the movements.

5. Focusing on basic skills and basic forms is not only important for beginners but also for high-level professional practitioners. Do not treat the basic training as a warm-up. That will not bring quality. For each training, we should set new and higher standards. For example, through the training of the basic steps of the Bagua Palm, we will make each step more fluid, more solid, and more stable with bigger range. Through the basic palm training, the palms will become better defined with clearer styles, such as the tuck-in palm, striking palm, piercing palm, and wiping palm, and each will be perfectly interpreted. For stance training, the twisting, wrapping, piercing, and turning of the body will be trained more prominently with very well-defined features. The basic skills and movements training do not have to be the same old story all the time. There are actually plenty of selections. We may tear them down flexibly and make the training more diversified and thus retain the interest of the trainees.

6. Pay great attention to the training of style, character, and mindset. Martial arts are not just about power and speed. Spirit, style, and expression are also very important, as well as the intrinsic character. Martial artists should have great self-confidence, a sense of brilliance, and the style of a gentleman. It all comes from the heart, as in the martial artist's old saying: "The mind follows the heart, *Qi* follows the mind, and the power comes with *Qi*." This tells us that everything comes from the heart. The martial artists should have not only an open mind but also a big heart and the manner of a hero. It is necessary to study traditional Chinese culture to enhance the self-cultivation process and learn more about the outstanding historical figures of China. All these will enable the trainees to love the Chinese martial arts more dearly and have better understanding of the core of martial arts.

7. Treat different people with different teaching styles. Tie the teaching method with the different talent and skill sets of each trainee. Everybody is different in terms of body, character, cognitive power, and ability in expressing themselves. So the teaching methods shall be tailored to the specialties and suit each person differently.

Part III: The Applications of Bagua Palm — Physically and Mentally

In Part I, we described what Bagua Palm is and the cultural soil from which it sprouted. In Part II, we introduced the way to practice Bagua Palm. In Part III, we will explain why we believe every single man and woman needs to learn some form of Bagua Palm.

It is not just something interesting to do.

It is the ideal exercise for every single person in our modern society. If you take the time you spend in practicing Bagua as an investment, it will deliver by far the biggest returns you could ever have.

Being busy is not an excuse not to learn Bagua; in fact, it is the reason why you should have learned it long ago. A real Bagua master integrates Bagua into everything he or she does. If you practice Bagua each day, you will not have to dedicate a single minute to doing any other physical exercises any more.

Let us find out why.

7
A Basic Conflict in Our Life:
How the Ultraslow Evolution of Our Body Cope with the Lightning-fast Changes of Our Environment

Recently, in the process of writing this book, I made a trip to a series of beautiful sea spots around the Cinque Terre in Italy (Fig. 7.1). As a reasonably strong amateur fighter and a semi-pro swimmer, I decided to swim in the rough sea and climb a steep rock for some fun.

I did make it, but I was almost smashed to pieces against the rocks by the furious waves, and I also found myself cut badly by sharp clam shells.

Pain is nothing for a fighter. The really bad thing was that for a while, I lost control of my own body. As the density of the human body is very close to that of sea water, I was perfectly carried by the gigantic waves to wherever it wanted me to go, at the pace set by the waves, which were not only fast but also unpredictable. It was like I was facing a far better fighter in the ring. That feeling was not a very comfortable one (Fig. 7.2).

Looking at my skin with hundreds of cuts, I realized how poorly protected I am as a human being from the forces of nature. We are not nearly as nimble as seals, and we do not have the skin of a shark or even a beaver.

Physically, we are not the strongest animal on this planet. Unlike previous dominant species on earth, we became dominant not because we are strong but because we are intelligent. We have not achieved our intelligence or dominance on this planet for very long. All the previous dominant species built their dominance on the bases of physical superiority, which was gained through hundreds of millions years of slow evolution, while we gained dominance with our relatively fast-developed intelligence. We changed the rules of the game.

Due to the capability of our brain, we not only created knowledge, but also created a medium to keep the knowledge, pass down the knowledge,

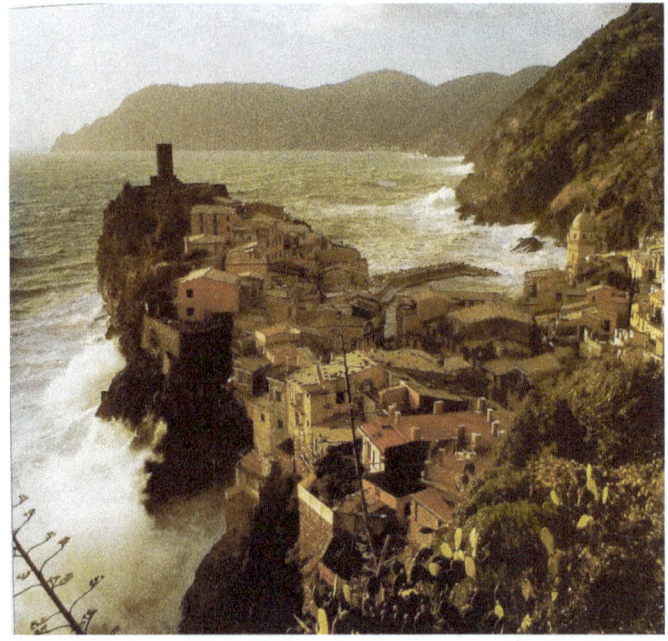

Fig. 7.1. The rough seas around Cinque Terre, Italy.

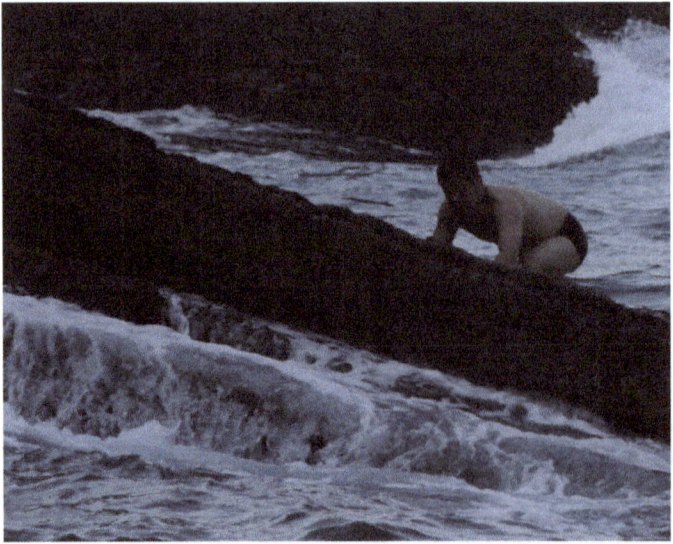

Fig. 7.2. I will not try this twice, not without a diving suit.

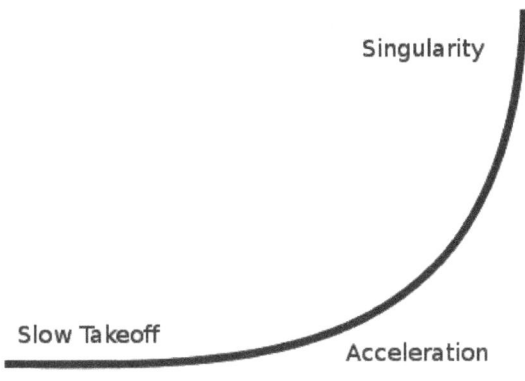

Fig. 7.3. Exponential growth curve.

and speed up the creation of future knowledge. This medium is called language. Because of language, the knowledge created by our ancestors never dies. What is more, when two pieces of knowledge are combined, a new piece of knowledge will be created.

A mathematician would describe the growth of our knowledge as an exponential growth curve. This is also the nature of how our environment changes, because we change our environment with our knowledge. The more knowledge we create, the faster we will change our environment by applying our knowledge.

We can see from Fig. 7.3 that initially the progress looks slow, but over a certain period of time, it accelerates suddenly and shoots to the sky, never turning back.

No wonder we have managed to dominate this planet so quickly. No wonder even we feel dizzy sometimes about the speed of change in the environment that we have created, especially when we observe the unbelievable progresses of our technology and the ever accelerating speed of environmental changes that affect our daily lives.

No wonder the Chinese legendary tale says that when words were created, the heavens rained down on crops and the ghosts cried in the night. Language is powerful. The growth rate of our knowledge is indeed awesome.

On the other hand, as we all know, the process of biological evolution is very steady and slow — and that is why it is called evolution. We may not know much about the mechanism of biological evolution, but we know it is slow. It looks something like Fig. 7.4.

Fig. 7.4. This curve is not from any data, only to show that the growth is slow with irregular directions.

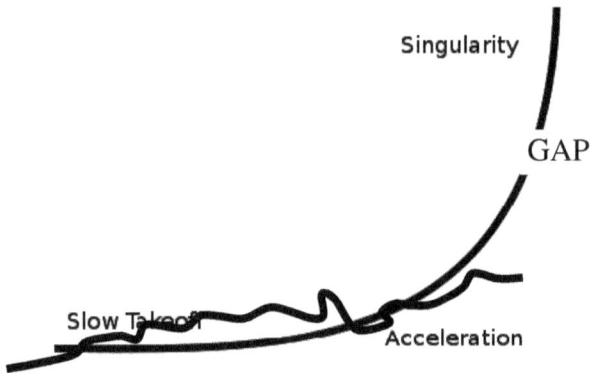

Fig. 7.5. The ever growing gap between our body and the environment.

It is not only slow, but it may not even have a set direction. There really is no guarantee that the line will even always go up. When we add these two curves together, we can see the real problem: the ever growing gap (Fig. 7.5).

This is the major source of the biggest conflict in our lives. On one hand, our environment changes at a dazzling speed, and the speed will accelerate even more due to the exponential nature of our knowledge acquisition; on the other hand, our physical body (and even a large part of our intangible soul) evolves at a very slow speed, close to zero, which never accelerates.

It is easy to figure out the seriousness of the problem: while the gap gets wider and wider, our body will find it more problematic to cope with the environment we have created.

Knowingly or not, with all the material improvement, we are creating a huge fundamental problem for ourselves. This problem will almost inevitably get bigger when we think we are making progress. Even if we fully understand what the problem is, there might not be any solution. This might not be an easy problem to tackle.

This problem is deadly intrinsic. The gap could grow forever, until the sharp conflict between our own body and the very environment we keep creating with our wisdom and hard work brings the whole history of mankind to an end.

This ever-growing gap will never be narrowed unless one of these two things happens:

1. We stop thinking, or
2. We develop some new method through genetic science to greatly accelerate our biological evolution and make it biological revolution.

The first option is unthinkable, while the second looks far from being even remotely possible.

This intrinsic conflict creates a paradox. We want to make progress all the time, and yet we want to pull back now, as we already feel uneasy about it. The very tool we have kept on developing to conquer the world ends up becoming the rock of Sisyphus. It seems impossible to solve such a problem.

Intrinsic conflicts always have the potential to drive people crazy, but maybe less so for the traditional Chinese who live it all the time. As we have mentioned, the Taoists believe conflicts are the sources of, or the drivers for, change. The Confucians, on the other hand, applied a middle-of-the-road strategy as a way of helping us face the unknown.

Following this line of thinking, we may choose to live in between the ancient and the modern, and stay alert for the necessary changes accordingly. We can obviously add back some ancient elements into our modern life without totally abandoning what we have achieved.

Of course we cannot simply go back to being cavemen and wait for our body's evolution to catch up. It is not even practical to choose an ancient activity to replace a modern one. Who wants to be a professional hunter today? However, it might be good to add back some ancient lifestyle elements as condiments, some typical elements of the ancient daily life, such as running and fighting, which have helped to shape our body as we see it today.

This is what we are suggesting here. It might be beneficial that all of us start to learn and practice fighting again. Some may find it hard to figure out the relevance of studying such an ancient art in a modern society, where most people are prosperous materially and well protected by law and order.

To understand exactly how this ancient art is relevant today, we need to go back and see where it comes from. I find two books are especially helpful to this topic: *The World Until Yesterday*[1] and *Sapiens: A Brief History of Humankind*.[2]

As we are the product of a slow evolution process, we are not much different from our ancestors, and it is always helpful to examine the factors that have helped in shaping what we are today.

Some research says people started to eat large quantities of meat about two million years ago. Not until about ten thousand years ago, the major source of food still came from gathering of fruits and hunting, which was basically running around and fighting with animals.[2] If there was nothing to hunt, people would need to fight with each other to get food for survival.

There is one thing I do not agree with the researchers in this field: the year *Homo sapiens* started to dominate the planet.

Evidence shows that large numbers of carnivore types started to diminish since about two million years ago, coinciding with the time *Homo sapiens* started consuming more meat. Many researchers believe it was due to starvation caused by food competition rather than direct killing by *Homo sapiens*. They think *Homo sapiens* was still physically too weak to fight with the larger types of carnivores.

They really do not understand fighting. Fighting with a weapon and barehanded are totally different things; weapon fighting relies more on the brain than physical power. As noted before, we changed the rules of the game with our brain. Barehanded, I may find it hard to fight against a lion. However, with a two-meter long bludgeon, I can handle any carnivore with proper training and practice.

Martial art practitioners have been dominating as individuals for far longer with their fighting skills. Martial art is never a pure physical art. It is an art of both wisdom and power, and you cannot even separate the two in fighting.

In the history of long evolution, which has slowly shaped our physical body, we had to be good fighters to survive, either fighting with animals or with other people. We were not designed to sit in front of a desk all day; we were not even designed to work in the field harvesting crops. We were designed by nature into a well-tuned fighting machine to kill for a living.

During the recent few thousand years, civilization has sped up dramatically. We kept livestock, and farming solved most of our food supply issues.

Ever since farming started 10,000 years ago, people began to have issues with their bodies, as we were not designed for those jobs like carrying heavy things and bending all day in a large crop field. It is natural that people's spines started to feel bad. However, we were still physically active then, and our bodies were stronger.

As time went on, things actually got better and worse at the same time.

Even less than 100 years ago, food was still a serious daily headache for normal people. The majority of people work very hard day in and day out just to feed themselves and their family members.

Look at where we are today. Normal people in civilized countries no longer worry about food. Even at midnight, there are shops open 24 hours every day, or even easier, we can open our refrigerator at home and get stuffed with all kinds of ready-to-eat food.

The dramatic lifestyle difference has resulted in our body looking very different. From pictures found in caves, people over 10,000 years ago looked much stronger in their legs. At the same time, they seemed to have much slimmer upper bodies (Fig. 7.6). In contrast, many people today have weaker legs and fatter bodies.

The differences make absolute sense, as we run much less and eat much more today compared with people over 10,000 years ago.

Ever if we do not judge which type of body shape is better, we can be pretty sure that our present shape does not match our existing body structure as well as in the past, because our organs do not have very different structures compared to 10,000 years ago.

Compare Fig. 7.6 with Fig. 7.7, which shows the cartoon of a 21st-century office worker.

We used to run a lot and eat little, but now the reverse is true. We used to sleep early and get up early, but now many people's sleeping habits are far from ideal. We used to spend a lot of time talking with each other, but now we stare all the time at a little screen.

Nowadays, even the real wars are no longer won by martial arts expertise. So, even as a self-defense skill, martial arts is no longer frequently needed, as the legal system does most of the work in keeping ordinary people safe.

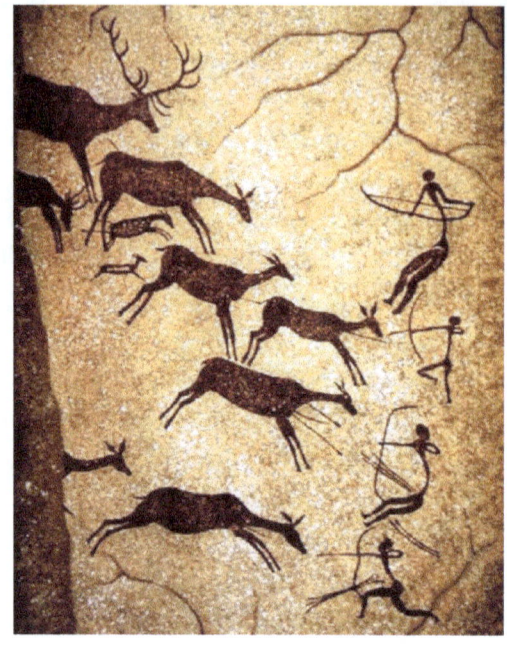

Fig. 7.6. Cave picture of hunters, 10,000 BC.

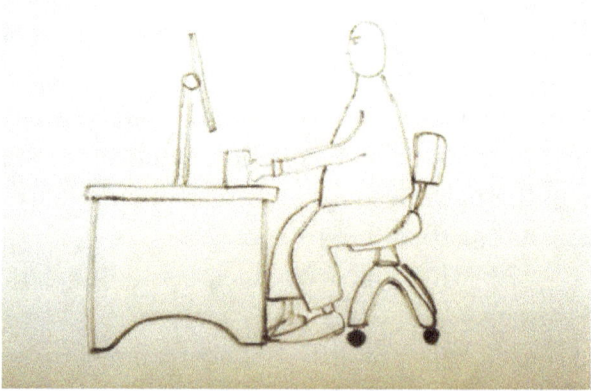

Fig. 7.7. A cartoon of a typical office worker today.

Fighting as an activity has almost been eliminated from our daily life.

As mentioned before, we were given a fighter's body over millions of years of evolution. In a mere hundreds of years, we stopped needing to fight any more. In the recent 30 years, we do not even need to move our body very often any more.

Does our body like this? Of course not. That is the major source of a relatively new group of diseases, called *lifestyle diseases*.

No wonder all types of so-called action movies have blockbuster movies. No wonder sports channels are so popular today. We are psychologically compensating ourselves for what our bodies are deprived of. This "compensation" not only tells us that the body needs to fight, but it also tells us that the body and mind are very closely connected, or as the Chinese martial arts classics puts it: "Body and mind as one."

This type of "compensation" is a common physical phenomenon. When people lose their eyesight, they begin to hear much better. Some armless people can use their feet to accomplish everything we do with our hands.

New research has even found that this type of "compensation" is also quite common in our brain. When one part of our brain is damaged, some other part will take over and compensate for the original functions of the lost part of the brain.[3]

Now we know that this type of "compensation" is also possible between our body and brain. This strengthens the belief that our body and mind are one. Just as the Chinese traditional medical practitioners believe that many diseases of our body originate from the mind and vice versa, Chinese martial artists believe the best way to be mentally strong is to strengthen ourselves physically and vice versa.

It is questionable whether the India monk — Bodhi dharma or *da* (达 reach) *mo* (摩 touch) was actually the founder of the outer school of Chinese martial arts. However, Bodhi dharma is unanimously regarded as the first master of Zen in China. The reason he is almost artificially claimed as the founder of Shaolin is more spiritual than operational. He was a master who promoted enlightenment through ascetic practice, which basically involved physical endurance of all kinds of pain.

People who talk about Bodhi dharma's Zen nowadays often focus on the sudden enlightenment part and forget about the long-term ascetic practice part, which is actually the very core of the outer school of Chinese martial arts. To strengthen ourselves, we need to involve both mind and body, as they are not separable.

The reason why we need to maximize the effect of strengthening ourselves, both physically and mentally, is that it is the only hope for us to cope with the unforeseeable future which is dominated by the intrinsic conflict between ourselves and the environment we keep creating.

Chinese martial art is thus relevant, not because martial art is a typical ancient activity, but also because it is a rare activity which involves both our body and mind intensively.

To effectively strengthen ourselves, we need first to truly understand the word *strong* and its meaning. I have found Nassim Taleb's book helpful in this regard. We will discuss this in the next chapter.

References

1. Jared Diamond (2013). *The World Until Yesterday: What Can We Learn from Traditional Societies?* Reprint Penguin Books.
2. Yuval Noah Harari (2015). *Sapiens: A Brief History of Humankind.* Harper edition, p. 87.
3. Norman Doidge (2015). *The Brain That Changes Itself*, 1st ed. Viking.

8
Anti-Fragile as a Concept and How Do We Understand "Strong"?

In his brilliant book, *Antifragile: Things That Gain from Disorder,* Nassim Nicholas Taleb argued convincingly that since the future is extremely difficult to predict, the best way to survive a disaster is not to try in vain to predict it but to strengthen ourselves and greatly increase our chances of survival when it actually happens in the unforeseeable future.[1]

The only thing I do not like is the word he used: *anti-fragile*. Taleb explains that anti-fragile is stronger than *strong*. Strong means not easily breakable. Anti-fragile means when struck, the object not only does not break but it also becomes even stronger than ever.

Taleb may be justified in creating this new word. However, I would rather use more friendly words for the same concept, even at the cost of semantic accuracy.

Anti-fragile as he defined it cannot be found in any inanimate material. Even the toughest material in the world does not have such a property. When struck, steel does not break easily, but it does not become stronger either. There might be some surface hardening, but it leads mostly to brittleness rather than toughness.

So, anti-fragile is mostly a property of living creatures.

Take the example of a Muay Thai fighter's shin: Muay Thai is a martial art from Thailand, where people are quite slight in build. So the Muay Thai fighters apply kicks and elbow jabs a lot more often than people trained in most other martial arts. One of their most feared weapons is their shins.

The Muay Thai fighters kick with their shins massively, a move which causes pain even by watching it. Countless practitioners with other martial art skills are destroyed by Muay Thai boxers' powerful shin kicks. Why do they have much stronger shins than the others? How do they make it? They train their shins by kicking them against banana trees. What does not break their shins makes their shins stronger.

Actually the powerful kicks do cause fractures in their shins, just as they would do to normal people. The trick is that these fractures are micro-fractures and can be healed over time simply with rest. The healing process of the micro-fractures induces more calcium into the bones and makes the shins stronger.

This is a typical example of anti-fragile: what is supposed to damage a living creature only ends up making it stronger than ever.

The opposite action to the Muay Thai kicking is to take antibiotics whenever a fever occurs. It may make us feel better in the short term, physically or psychologically. But in the long run, this makes us even more vulnerable when faced with new viruses.

A sociology research in China on the descendants of the high-ranking officials of the late Qing Dynasty had results that aligned with the concept of anti-fragile. It found that those who had earned a lot of money from their position and left it to their children all saw their children spending all the money.

On the other hand, those who treated their children sternly and left practically no assets to them, mostly had children who became very successful scientists, artists, or diplomats.

As the pace of modern life increases, we may experience more good and bad things in our lives than our forebears did. This demands greater capability from us than from our ancestors to be anti-fragile. Ironically, as we live in a seemingly more pampered world, our anti-fragile capability is actually weaker compared with our ancestors who led much tougher lives.

We do not even have to look that far. In a recent outdoor activity organized by our company, we saw a peculiar line of people climbing a small hill: the eldest employees were far ahead, the middle-aged in the middle, and the youngsters were all far behind trying to catch their breath.

The formation of anti-fragile capability actually includes a negative feedback regulation mechanism.

Take the example of our body temperature while jogging. When our body temperature rises, our nerve system will detect it and a message will be sent to our brain. Then the temperature regulation center of our brain will react by sending instructions to the body to sweat. We will soon sweat all over, and our body temperature will be brought down.

The mechanism is called negative feedback regulation because it reacts to the disturbance of the stability of the system by a feedback that reverses the effects of the disturbance.

As we can observe from martial art training experiences, as with any other capabilities, the negative feedback mechanism has a very positive influence on self-healing capability. Self-healing is also a capability that can be enhanced over time with frequent exercises. In ancient times, the fighting was more dangerous than what we see today. As medical care barely existed, a simple wound could lead to death if the body could not heal itself.

Today, even with sophisticated methods to treat the wounds, martial arts are still widely regarded by the public as a dangerous sport. The fact is that the opposite is true. Not getting yourself involved in any martial art training is a dangerous decision. You not only risk yourself by losing anti-fragile capability when external disturbance occurs, but you also lose the benefit of getting hurt, when the hurt-induced micro-fractures could have greatly strengthened your bones.

The greatest and more indispensable benefit from martial art training is mental strength. Not just because mental strength is more important in modern life, but also because present medical science does a much poorer job in taking care of people's mental health than physical diseases.

What we actually see in a martial artist is real strength, which is a vivid spirit in a strong body. The redefined "strong" is not just the ability to sustain a hurt, but more, the anti-fragile capability to become stronger after getting hurt, both physically and mentally.

References

1. Nassim Nicholas Taleb (2012). *Antifragile : Things that gain from disorder.* New York: Random House.

9
Outlive as a Target and the Martial Art Renaissance

We introduced Taoism and Confucianism at the very beginning of the book for a good reason. Taoism together with Confucianism, which started almost at the same period in Chinese history, preached one thing in common — to go back to the ancient way of living. This looked absurd to the people who were intent on progress, and was even regarded as reactionary in some circles.

Now we can understand why it happened in that way during that period of time. That was the time when the Chinese started to have much greater productivity, and hence faced greater changes in social and economic areas. The tension caused by these changes became more than they could psychologically and physically handle.

Lao Zi and Confucius both observed those changes and understood the key problem: what was newer was not necessarily better. Both of them very sharply pointed out the solution, which was to learn from the previous generations and include some ancient elements into the new way of life.

Taoism and Confucianism offer the philosophical guidance for all Chinese martial arts. Therefore, through martial arts training, we can understand the philosophy more deeply.

As we have seen, it might be academically difficult to understand the reason for following the middle-of-the-road philosophy; however, from the perspective of martial artists, this position is very significant. In actual fighting, the most viable positioning is to stay in the middle, because we do not know what is going to happen. Staying in the middle gives us maximum options in uncertain situations. So when you do not know what is going to happen, stay in the middle.

Barely 10–20 years ago, the whole world was still enamored with the prosperity that modern science and technology have brought us. Old-time philosophies like Taoism and Confucianism did not have the capability to touch most people's hearts.

Now, things are starting to change. It seems we are reaching a tipping point where we suddenly find that Taoism and Confucianism may be relevant in our modern lives after all.

As people live longer, more and more people are concerned about healthcare and wellness issues. The medical resources of the more developed countries will continue to get tighter and tighter. This is a classic demand and supply issue.

People used to live till 75 years, now it maybe 85, and it can easily reach 95 by the end of 2020. The demand for medical care has already doubled and may triple by the end of 2020.

How about the story from the supply side? The growth is very liner if not declining. Only the smartest students will be accepted by medical schools, and not all the smart students want to go as they can easily find a decent life elsewhere. No matter how the situation goes, the number of doctors is not going to double or triple any time soon.

The intrinsic conflict between demand and supply only points to one direction: in a purely rational and monopolistic market, the prices will go up. The actual situation might be worse than a price hike, with the riches of the developing countries looking to the west for medical care.

It is only natural that we are concerned about the future of the elderly. It is more natural that all of us start to spend more time on all kinds of exercises today. It is not even about living longer. It is about living with a higher quality of life, long after we retire.

If we apply the methodology of backward thinking to look for the sports that our ancestors engaged in the most, two would definitely stand out. Among all the sports, running and fighting were the most frequent physical activities for our ancestors.

Firstly, let us look at running as the most popular way of exercising today. The early *Homo sapiens*, our closest forebears, used to run nonstop for hours until the animals they were hunting fell because of heat exhaustion. Our ancestors got to eat not because they were faster or stronger than the animals, but because they could run and sweat at the same time. The animals they hunted had to stop frequently to cool themselves off.

So we are great long-range runners by design. We used to run a great deal.

Running is obviously a great sport today as well, but we need to be careful about the difference between modern running and pre-historical running. The difference is not complicated — it is the running shoes that we wear. We now have running shoes when we used to run with bare feet.

The first significant difference is the force we apply when we push off. Without a pair of running shoes, we are much more careful and almost never apply too much force, thus our knees will be much less impacted.

The second difference is that when we run with bare feet, to further lessen the impact and protect our feet from sharp objects on the ground, we were very careful when stepping down. We used to lift our front legs with the help of our abs, and step down tentatively without committing our body weight. Only when we were sure that it was safe, did we move our body weight to the front leg.

This whole process of ancient walking or running is very similar to the mud-wading steps we practice in Bagua forms. Those moves not only strengthen our abs, but also massage the organs behind our abs for better blood circulation inside those organs.

The third difference is that, because there were no roads and no shoes, every step was different for the ancient runners. I have to admit that I think the ancient runners had much more fun and much less chance of getting hurt because running was not a highly repetitive activity then.

As we all know, human tissues are very easily worn out with repetitive impacts. In that sense, a martial art poses a far better type of exercise, as it has so many forms and you never have to repeat any form if you do not want to.

On the other hand, martial art principles can be internalized over a period of time. After that, even if you are not training, you are doing it whenever you make a move. Whether in opening a door, brushing your teeth, or even raising your hand to say hello to somebody, you are moving with the martial art rules applied.

That is the beauty of practicing martial arts, which no other sport possesses. If you are not playing football, you are not playing football; if you are not running, you are not running; whereas if you are not practicing Chinese martial arts, you are still doing it all the time!

Chinese martial arts, once you are trained in it, functions like a legendary Chinese protection dragon who always follows you wherever you go, protecting you all the way.

As the latest traditional Chinese martial arts ever formed by the best fighter in the late Qing Dynasty, Bagua is actually the ultimate martial arts. It is not just scientific, but also beautiful. Like running, it involves a lot of footwork, so the biggest muscle group in your body gets trained. Like Yoga, it trains not only your body but also your mind and your soul. It brings peace into your life.

At the same time, Bagua does have powerful self-defense applications. It is like a running Yoga with fighting applications. It is such a complete sport.

I believe that Bagua has the potential to become the most practiced form of Chinese martial arts eventually, as it is easier to teach and practice with proper adjustment to help people learn step by step, literally.

It is one of the best candidates to be added as an ingredient to the fast-paced daily life of normal people in modern society.

With *Jing* and *Yi* obtained from Bagua training, we are beyond antifragile. We will be able to gain great vitality, which is actually the biggest difference between a human being and a pile of mud. We will be truly on the top of the vitality rankings, which can be demonstrated in a sequence as mud, plant, sheep, wolf, and human beings.

Vitality as the capability to change is a great tool for the small to beat the giant. Even in the business world, smaller companies with great vitality, and thus, great capability and willingness to change, always beat those giant companies with weak vitality.

In ancient times, fighting is everyone's task and it was thus in the genes of our body. Martial arts used to be mastered by all people. About 5000 years ago, it became a highly specialized skill and dropped out of normal people's life. In about 150 years ago, with the sophistication of guns, it lost its position in society. Now, we have found it again, in times of great change.

The environment is still challenging and unpredictable. However, trained martial artists are never that anxious. They just take the best position and stay alert. Their well-trained ability to change abruptly and their experiences in actual fighting brings them a solid feeling of security, which leads to calmness and unique charm. That is what martial arts can give us, mentally and physically.

As more and more people start to understand the value of Chinese martial arts, there is going to be another great Renaissance in history: the Martial Art Renaissance.

This I so declare.

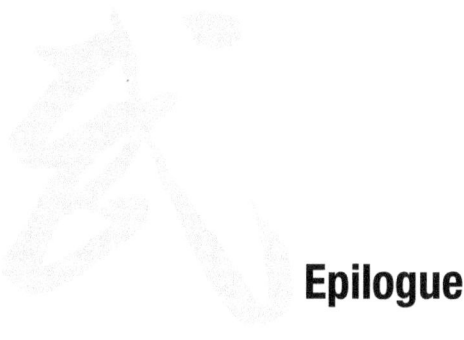

Epilogue

水落石出
— The rock appears when the water level falls.

This is a book about martial arts. And yet, this is not a book solely about martial arts, because martial arts is not all about martial arts. Given the important role it played in civilization, it is an indispensable part of culture.

Now we have entered a tricky area. With the exchange of ideas happening all the time, each nation still has its own unique piece of culture developed in a relatively closed environment over hundreds, if not thousands, of years. And there is a lot of pride involved. To say the least, there is a big gap between the eastern and western cultures. And conflicts happen.

For example, while reading this book, the Chinese may feel bewildered by so many "non-poetic" physics concepts applied to interpret an elegant ancient art. The westerners, on the other hand, may read in disbelief and think the whole Chinese martial arts thing is just a myth, not reality. We do not see many successful Chinese fighters in either boxing or mixed martial arts (MMA) fields, anyway.

As a Chinese, I am not even qualified to play the judge on which culture is superior. There is a lot of heat, especially in China, in the debate over whether the Chinese culture is just inferior as a whole to that of western society. The attempt to put the Chinese culture in a place to compete with the whole western culture is a joke from the beginning, as Chinese culture was never in such a place even at its peak.

In order not to make this epilogue another book, I would like to end these types of disputes with one larger view. Human beings existed on this planet for at least a few millions of years. It was only less than 5000 years ago that knowledge began to grow rapidly. And modern science emerged less than 500 years ago. We are still in the very beginning of a knowledge explosion. It is just too early to judge who has the best way.

So should we preserve the "purity" of each other's culture or should we mix them all up and get the best for ourselves? The answer is: it depends.

Each person may choose to play different roles in their own lives or in different parts of their lives. If you would like to devote yourself as a scholar to preserve a distinct culture, there is a place for you in this world. If you choose to be a fighter, you have to get the best suitable weapon for yourself. You have to have the best weapon just to survive.

It does not have to be the No. 1 ranked weapon in the world, but it has to suit you, because you are part of the weapon. It does not work if you and your weapon do not get along.

You may even have to break all the existing weapons and forge one for yourself. That is the approach of this book — a fighter's approach. We take the necessary elements of different cultures and make ourselves a true lethal weapon from them.

This book is not for you to keep on your bookshelf. We do not even have the intention for you to remember anything this book tells you. What we want is for you to start practicing, to experience what was said in this book with your body and mind, to internalize this book and make it become an integral part of you, so that you do not have to remember anything. The time you forget about everything in this book is the time we can claim success as writers.

When you start learning martial arts, you become a fighter in the making. In the long process of becoming a better fighter, there is pain, frustration, and ultimately, joy. You will not regret it unless you give up. So never, never, never give up. That is the reason for the strong words from Churchill: Never, never, never, never, never give up.

Now we are all fighters. At least in our minds we are, as we have finished this book together.

Congratulations, and move on!

Acknowledgments

This is not a typical martial arts book.

The major portion of the book was written by Master Li Jun Feng in Chapter 6, with the pictures of the forms taken of Master Ge Chun Yan's performance. The actual work was done with the efforts from many grand masters during the golden years of Chinese martial arts — the 1980s. That was the time when numerous true masters of Chinese martial arts were practicing in Beijing, including Master Li Jun Feng and his teachers, while the young athletes then, such as Master Ge Chun Yan, were very dedicated to learning and practicing without the distraction of material abundance. Such coincidence will probably not happen again.

Chapter 5 is the summary of Master Ge Chun Yan's unique training method.

The rest of the chapters were written by Luo Tong, including the translations as the original manuscript of Chapters 5 and 6 were in Chinese. Luo Tong would like to thank the Physics Department of Peking University, and especially his physics teacher in Suzhou Middle School, Mr. Wang Yi Ran, for imparting him with solid education and love for science in general.

The original paintings in Figs. 1.1, 1.5, 1.6, 2.1, and 2.2 are from the art works of Ms. Mao Ying, who as an art enthusiast, used to work with Simpson Thacher & Bartlett LLP and met many inspiring people on and off the job.

www.ingramcontent.com/pod-product-compliance
Lightning Source LLC
Chambersburg PA
CBHW081348230426
43667CB00017B/2765